Ketogenic Diet

Do's and Don'ts for Rapid Weight Loss

I0428903

Collin Dowling

Introduction

I want to thank you and congratulate you for downloading the book, *"Ketogenic Diet, Dos and Don'ts for Rapid Weight Loss."*

Everyone wants to lose weight quickly, but the real issue is how to do so safely. Completely removing specific food groups from daily meals, and severely limiting calorie intake may lead to dramatic weight loss, but it can seriously compromise the health of your internal organs, which could lead to multiple and serious health complications down the line. In worse case scenarios, this could lead to permanent kidney damage, liver failure, and even cardiac arrest.

The most common and irritating consequence of dramatic weight loss is the body's insistence to regain all those excess pounds. It may even insist on adding more for good measure – a condition called yo-yo dieting. This makes slimming down such a Herculean task.

Unlike other diets, Ketogenic diet encourages consumption of less carbohydrates, but higher levels of fat. Although this may sound counterintuitive, especially in terms of losing weight quickly, this eating regimen works well for people who have struggled with their weight all their lives, or those who are prone to yo-yo dieting.

Ketogenic diet works on the principle that a body in a state of **ketosis** can burn off more stored fat in the adipose tissues. When done properly, this leads to gradual but safe weight loss. It also makes weight management easier to do afterwards, which basically eliminates yo-yo dieting.

This book contains information on how to follow the Ketogenic diet correctly and more importantly: gradually and safely. Make no mistake about it. This is a rigorous and exacting eating regimen that entails solid preparation beforehand. Aside from containing basic guidelines for the diet, tips on meal planning and list of specific food items to consume and avoid, this book also contains easy-to-follow recipes that novice cooks can make in their kitchen.

There is also a 3-month (90-day) meal plan sample to start you off in your Ketogenic diet.

Thanks again for downloading this book. I hope you enjoy it!

Table of Contents

Chapter 1: Truth You Need to Know About Carbohydrates

When a person consumes food and drink, the gastric system automatically breaks these down into macronutrients -- ideally, into glucose, lipids (fats) and proteins, which blood can easily absorb and transport into different organs of the body. Glucose is the brain's main food supply. This is extracted from carbohydrates.

In the past decade or so, carbohydrates gained a lot of bad reputation. Celiac disease aside, many people unjustly branded this as something to avoid at all cost. It became target for numerous gastric diseases, respiratory ailments, skin problems, and of course, weight gain.

Truth is: this food group is not inherently bad for one's health. Consuming good carbs or complex carbohydrates helps regulate mood, improves mental/memory functions, promotes restive sleep, provides good sources of fiber (that aids bowel movement and organic removal of toxins,) and elevates your energy to get you through the day.

Food items classified as complex carbohydrates are usually plant-based. Because many of these are consumed with their rigid plant cells intact (also termed "whole"), the body's gastric system digests these at a slow rate. This leaves the person feeling full for longer periods of time, which is a valuable aid to weight management. Rigid cells in plant matter absorb soluble fiber, which clears the way for insoluble fiber to absorb as much toxins in the bloodstream, and expels these out of the body.

Examples of complex carbohydrates are: fresh fruits and vegetables, dried or fresh pulses (beans, legumes, lentils, soy, etc.,) dairy (low fat yogurt, skim milk, etc.), nuts, seeds, and whole grains (barley, buckwheat, corn, dark-colored rice, slow cooking oats, sorghum, whole wheat, whole grains, etc.)

The real issue here is the person's daily intake of simple carbohydrates. As the name suggests, these contain simple starches/sugars that the blood cells readily absorb. Some of these go through the entire circulatory and gastric systems without being properly digested. Simple carbs contains loose molecules that easily pass through stomach walls and almost instantaneously become blood sugar.

An increase in blood sugar level forces the pancreas to produce more hormones, called insulin, to break these down into glucose. Unfortunately, when blood becomes overly saturated with sugar, the pancreas produces poor quality or quantity of insulin that becomes ineffective in its role. This is a condition called **insulin resistance**.

This is commonly seen in people with diabetes. Type I diabetics do not produce enough insulin in their bodies, while Type II diabetics produce high volumes of insulin that cannot break down sugars in the bloodstream.

Chronic episodes of insulin resistance become a metabolic downward spiral. When unmanaged, sugar stays in the bloodstream without being converted into glucose – the brain's primary source of nutrition. When this happens, the brain undergoes the first stages of nutritional "starvation."

It sends out panic signals to the rest of the body that it needs to consume carbs that can easily be converted into glucose, specifically: sugary food items and beverages. This is a condition called **sweet tooth syndrome**.

At one point in our lives, we may have experienced this. This manifests when we crave for sweets after heavy meals, or when we don't content ourselves from consuming single portions of carbohydrate-rich food and drinks (e.g. cake, candies, sodas, etc.), or when we suddenly crave for specific food items out of the blue, especially for greasy and salty food, (as these usually have high carbohydrate content too.)

However, because the body is already in a state of insulin resistance, consuming carbs only starves the brain further. The relentless panic signals intensify.

These signals include, but are not limited to: the urge to keep eating even when you are full (overindulgence,) addiction to sugar-rich beverages or candies, and even midnight snacking (the urge to eat hours after dinner, usually in between sleeping time.)

One of the worst things about insulin resistance is bad diet and sedentary lifestyle can easily trigger it. It needs a restrictive eating regimen, and sometimes, medical intervention to stop it from happening on a regular basis.

In this time and age, it is easy to overindulge in simple carbohydrates. Even if you are trying to eat "healthy" meals, these can creep up on you in unexpected ways.

These are in:

- **ALL** forms of sweeteners, organic and man-made. There is no escaping the fact that sweeteners **ARE** simple carbs. It doesn't matter what kind you use, the moment you consume these, their molecules immediately break down into simple starches, which pass through stomach linings and into the bloodstream. Consuming the smallest amount drastically affects insulin production in the pancreas.

  Sweeteners may be in your breakfast drinks, in your granola bars, and in your salad dressings. It is definitely in your glass of wine, in your sports drink, and in that cup of low-fat yogurt you eat as snacks.

  Canned spaghetti sauces, barbeque flavored meat-based dinners, and even potato chips are food products that you never think of containing sugar, but these have the highest amounts -- up to 4 to 6 teaspoons of sweeteners per single serving.

  Different kinds of sweeteners include, but are not limited to:*

  - Acesulfame K (A)
  - Advantame (A)
  - Agave syrup (M)
  - Aspartame (A)
  - Barley Malt Syrup (M)
  - Birch Syrup (SE)
  - Brazzein (NS)
  - Brown Rice Syrup (M)
  - Cane Juice (SE)
  - Caramel (M)
  - Coconut Palm Sugar (SE)
  - Corn Sugar/Syrup (M)

- Dextrose (PS)
- Fructose (PS)
- Galactose (PS)
- Glucose (PS)
- Golden Syrup (M)

* Legend: A – Artificial or man-made sweeteners, M – modified tar extract, NS – natural sweeteners, PS – pure or natural sugar, SE – sugar extract, SF – sugar fiber

- Honey (PS)
- Inulin (SF)
- Inverted sugar (M)
- Lactose (PS)
- Maltodextrin (PS)
- Maltose (PS)
- Maple Syrup (SE)
- Miraculin (NS)
- Molasses (SE)
- Neotame (A)
- Palm Sugar (SE)
- Rapadura (SE)
- Refiner's Sugar/Syrup (M)
- Saccharin (A)
- Sorghum Syrup (SE)
- Stevia (NS)
- Sucralose (A)
- Sucrose (PS)
- Yacon Syrup (NS)

- Fortified or white grains, and all food items/drinks that contain these, e.g.

  - Overly refined grains

    - Breakfast cereals, mostly processed corn and wheat

- Breakfast drinks that contain corn or oats or other grains
- Oats, instant and/or quick cooking

o Commercial pasta, all kinds

o Easy-to-cook meat products (these use refined starches to extend meat)

- Chicken nuggets, frozen, ready-to-cook
- Hotdogs and canned sausages
- Frozen or canned meat, including diet food/meals/snacks
- Pre-marinated meat

o White flour

- Cake mixes, ready-made or ready-to-bake/steam
- Commercially produced breads, cakes, cookies, pastries, other baked goods
- Commercial condiment, gravies, sauces and soups
- Frozen bread and/or dough
- Frozen, boxed, packed, or ready-to-eat desserts

o White rice

- Ready-to-cook/frozen rice desserts and meals
- Microwave or quick cooking rice
- Microwave or quick cooking congee

- Processed food and beverages, all kinds. These contain sweeteners and overly refined starches, not to mention harmful food additives and preservatives.

So, where do all these carbs go if these are not converted into glucose?

In ideal situations, when a person consumes too much of anything, the gastric system does its best to expel these out of the body in the quickest way possible. It can go out via bowel movement, sweating or urination. Or, in the case of overindulgence of alcohol and/or dairy products, these are sometimes expelled through vomiting. Expelling food quickly, even violently stabilizes blood sugar levels and insulin production.

When someone is in the throes of insulin resistance, and amidst the brain's relentless panic signals, the body instinctively hoards all forms of calories into adipose tissues that are essentially fat cells. Then it creates more adipose tissues so that it can keep on hoarding. This is the body's way of preserving itself amidst perceived but not-existent "starvation."

Hoarding in this case also means preventing the body from releasing these stored calories. This is basically why it is difficult to lose weight in the first place. Often, this form of cellular hoarding goes out of hand, and the body cannot produce enough adipose tissues any more. Unprocessed calories (in the form of lipids) are then deposited as plaques in arteries and veins, which the body ignores or refuses to expel.

This leads to mental confusion, slower metabolism, lethargy, inexplicable exhaustion, higher susceptibility to bone, ligament or tendon damage, higher risks of bacterial, fungal, or viral infections, and of course, uncontrollable weight gain.

Chapter 2: Benefits of Following Ketogenic Diet

Ketogenic diet is a restrictive diet. Designed initially to ease some symptoms of refractory epilepsy in children under the age of 12, this eating regimen promotes consumption of small amounts of complex carbohydrates, with moderate amounts of protein, but unlike other diets, this entails eating food items high in fat.

Ideally, when a person consumes fatty/oily food, the liver produces higher volumes of ketone bodies: water-soluble molecules that can break down fat/oil, so that nutrients are extracted, and the rest are processed out of the body immediately. This produces energy (calories) that is not dependent on glucose in the bloodstream.

The Ketogenic diet works with this principle in mind.

It encourages minimal carbohydrate intake, with high fat consumption so that the body undergoes **ketosis**. This is a physiological state wherein the body relies on ketone bodies to produce nutritional sustenance for internal organs.

What are the benefits?

Because the brain still needs glucose in order to function properly, it starts using hoarded calories in adipose tissues that are ignored during insulin resistance. It is only during this time when the brain finally stops sending out panic signals to the rest of the body. This lessens frequency and intensity of food cravings and in many cases, even reduces or controls appetite naturally.

Less carbohydrates in the bloodstream promotes better **insulin sensitivity** – a condition wherein the pancreas produces better quality and quantity of insulin hormones that processes starches/sugars better. This is the complete opposite of **insulin resistance**.

For people who are chronically overweight and/or obese for a long time, who with all probability also suffer from NAFLD (non-alcoholic fatty liver disease,) entering a state of ketosis can remove, limit, and in the future, prevent fatty buildup in the liver. This makes kidneys, circulatory system, and gastric system function well.

Moderate consumption of protein while on the Ketogenic diet preserves and improves the health of muscles, bones, ligaments and tendons.

This leads to organic, gradual but safe weight loss.

Other advantages of Ketogenic diet include:

1. It burns off almost all stored energy in the body, with very little negative repercussions on the rest of the internal organs.

    Other restrictive diets discourage the consumption of one or more food groups like carbohydrates and fats. Although these diets yield rapid weight loss, it seriously compromises major internal organs.

    For example: diets that severely restrict carbohydrate-intake contribute to brain "starvation" or hypoglycemia. This leads to mental fogginess, premature memory loss, and in extreme cases, even onset of mild dementia and other mental disorders. Other complications may include: anxiety, chills (uncontrollable bodily shaking,) depression, double vision, chronic exhaustion, fainting spells, heart palpitations, nausea, physical lethargy, sweating, and overall weakness.

For people with Type II diabetes, hypoglycemia can lead to diabetic coma (due to low blood sugar,) and without medical intervention, even early demise.

Diets that severely restrict fat/oil-consumption contribute to: hair loss, premature skin aging, and yellowing/chipped nails. Liver and nerve tissues of the brain need a healthy supply of fats in order to function properly.

The body also needs this particular food group to absorb fat-soluble nutrients like: Vitamins A, D, E and K. Without these, a person may suffer from: anemia, ataxia (chronic loss of balance,) bleeding gums, premature bone loss, chapped/cracked lips, deep muscle pain, dry eyes, headaches, heavy monthly bleeding (for women in child-bearing years,) infertility, joint pains, nose bleeds, premature blindness, and progressive retinal damage.

The risk of acquiring certain diseases rises exponentially, too. These include: cancer, cardiovascular diseases, Crohn's disease, ED or erectile dysfunction, glucose intolerance, hypertension, inflammatory bowel disease, multiple sclerosis and peripheral neuropathy (permanent nerve damage to hands/feet increase.)

2. You don't feel hungry all the time.

Some diets, especially those that promote ready-made frozen dinners/meals and snacks contain too few calories, but high amounts of sugar, food additives and preservatives. This leaves the person feeling hungry all the time.

Many people mistakenly believe that hunger is a good thing when dieting. This is the farthest thing from the truth.

Hunger makes you think of food all the time. During unguarded moments, it makes you want to cheat on your diet constantly. Sometimes, it even encourages you to binge heavily on greasy, salty and sugary food items and drinks at the first opportunity.

One of the best things about the Ketogenic diet is that it suppresses appetite organically. This prevents or lessens risk of bingeing and overindulging.

3. For women, the Ketogenic diet promotes regular menstruation.

Other diets are so restrictive that vital nutrients like iron are removed entirely from the equation. For men, this has little or no consequences. However, for women of child bearing years, this greatly affects menstrual cycle.

With little or no iron in the diet, women tend to bruise easily, feel nauseous all the time, and suffer from intense or prolonged menstrual cramps. Some women report too frequent bleeding (twice or thrice a month,) while others report that their cycles stop or become erratic for the entire duration of the diet.

These can cause hair loss, infertility, numerous skin conditions (e.g. acne outbreak, enlarged pores, epidermal abrasions, flaky skin, skin discoloration, etc.), and in extreme cases, may also cause miscarriage.

4. Lastly, this diet is good for core muscles.

Many people go on restrictive diets to lose weight, but many of these neglect the health of core muscles. This makes them look lean and fit, but have very little energy for exercise or daily physical activities. This is often due to the body's prolonged "starvation" of one or more essential macronutrients like: carbohydrate, fats and proteins.

The Ketogenic diet promotes consuming all three macronutrients in specific amounts that will not only safeguard the health of core muscles and bones (from proteins,) but will also promote mental health (from carbs,) and integumentary/ nerve health (from fats.)

Good core muscles also contribute to speedy weight loss, as these are the ones that can burn off calories the fastest.

Chapter 3: How to Get Started with the Keto Diet

This is a restrictive and exacting diet. This is the first thing you need to know about this eating regimen. Aside from consuming particular food groups in specific amounts, you should also know that any slip-up (e.g. incorrect proportions of carbs-fat-protein intake) can set you back very quickly.

Not only do you need detailed meal plans, but counting calories is also a must.

Other things you need to know about the Keto Diet are:

1. This is not for everyone.

    People with certain medical and physical conditions are discouraged from following this diet, like:

    - People with existing cardiovascular diseases. Any restrictive diet taxes the brain and the heart – two major organs that are highly dependent on blood flow. Those who are taking powerful medications for heart ailments and high blood pressure are discouraged from following the Ketogenic diet.

      The same holds true for people who already suffered from stroke, had one or more forms of cardiac surgeries, and those who had (or about to undergo) brain surgery.

    - People with gallbladder diseases, or those who had surgical procedures to remove gallbladder. Without this (or with a malfunctioning) organ, the body cannot metabolize all forms of fat or lipids. The person needs to take additional medications and food supplements to sustain good health. This condition paired with Keto diet can tax the person's liver and kidneys further, which can lead to serious health repercussions like blood poisoning and renal failure.

- People with inflammatory bowel disorders (IBD,) like: Crohn's disease and ulcerative colitis. This can trigger or prolong painful cramps and intensify inflammation of the digestive tract, which could lead to multiple infections.

The same is true for people with rare metabolic disorders like: Fabry disease, Friedreich ataxia, Galactosemia, Gaucher disease, Glycogen storage disease, Hurler syndrome, Krabbe disease, maple syrup urine disease, mitochondrial disorder, Niemann-Pick disease, Tay-Sachs disease, etc. which could interfere with fat oxidation.

- People who take powerful medications for anxiety, depression, or other forms of psychological disorders. These medications can negatively affect the person's ability to properly process toxins out of the body. The Ketogenic diet promotes massive flushing of toxins from the body through urination and sweat.

Unfortunately, lithium and similar drugs need to slowly metabolize in water to become effective. With water moving quickly out of the body, these drugs can stay in concentrated amounts in the blood, which can lead to poisoning.

- Pregnant and breastfeeding women, children under the age of 16, elderly people, people who recently undergone (or will undergo) any form of surgery, and people who are currently underweight, including anorexics. They all need higher than normal protein requirement. Subjecting them to Keto diet will only cause the onset of numerous gastrointestinal problems.

  For pregnant women, this increases risks of miscarriage or premature delivery. For breastfeeding women, this can cause milk to stop flowing, or can cause swelling of mammary glands, which can lead to infection.

- Type I diabetics, particularly those who regularly inject insulin. The Keto diet may cause dramatic insulin imbalance. Combined with medication (or lack thereof,) may lead to diabetic coma.

  Some reports show that these can be safely used by Type II diabetics, when supervised by health care providers.

2. You need the approval and/or supervision of a health care practitioner while on this diet.

   Even if you are at your fittest, you should never take this diet lightly. In the first few days, some people feel nauseous and weak. Many give up on the diet after only a couple of days, especially when they see how difficult it is to maintain the diet. This may be due to poor meal planning or not following the recommended macronutrient portions per meal.

If possible, ask a nutritionist or dietician to supervise your progress, especially if you have specific dietary preferences (e.g. vegan, vegetarian, etc.) or you are undergoing progressive training (e.g. body building, strength training, etc.) or you have any existing medical condition and/or taking powerful medications (e.g. Type II diabetes.)

3. Never combine Keto diet with other diets.

   If you are already following a different diet, it is highly recommended to stop the previous one, and allow your body to "rest" for at least 2 weeks. This doesn't mean that you should gorge on food, but it is essential that you stop taking supplements or drugs from your earlier diet, if any.

   Drink lots of water during this time, and plan your meals way in advance.

4. Buy Keto Sticks.

   These are readily available in most drug stores. If these are not on the shelves, ask the pharmacist to order some for you before you start your diet, or you can always buy several boxes online.

   Keto sticks indicate if your body is in the state of ketosis. All you have to do is dab one piece in your morning urine. The moistened area changes color accordingly. Normally, when the stick turns:

   - Green – This means that your body is in the state of ketosis. You are consuming low volumes of carbohydrates, and high amounts of good fats, and enough protein to sustain good health.

- Blue – Your body is still in the state of ketosis. You are still consuming low volumes of carbohydrates, but you need to increase your good fat and protein intake slightly.

- Orange – Your body is almost nearly out of the ketosis stage. Your carbohydrate intake is higher than the recommended amount, and your good fat and protein intake is low.

- Red – Your body is no longer in the state of ketosis. Your carbohydrate and protein intake are high, but your good fat intake is low. Once you reach this stage, you need to do the Keto diet over, which may take another 2 days to 3 weeks.

Common Mistakes People Make When Following the Keto Diet

1. Making meal plans without the approval or supervision of a health care provider.

   People have individual dietary needs and different lifestyles. Although you can undertake this task by yourself, you should always remember that one small slip up can delay **ketosis.** This is the state you need to achieve in order to burn off as much stored calories as possible.

   When properly done, a person can achieve ketosis in as little as 2 days. Any mistake in food planning can delay this state by as much as 3 weeks.

   If possible, work with a registered dietician (or sports nutritionist, if you are actively working out,) during the first week of your Keto diet.

   Or, at the very least, go to your doctor and ask for a full check-up. Have your blood sugar and insulin levels checked. More importantly, if you are taking powerful medications as treatment for any condition, ask your health care provider if you can work around these so you can lose weight safely.

2. Making meals on the fly.

   Always plan, and if possible, make your meals in advance. Counting calories for each meal can become a tedious task, especially for first time Keto dieters. A hectic lifestyle, and/or unexpected events (e.g. emergency trip to the hospital,) can further complicate the situation. If you don't plan ahead, it is easy to miscalculate your macronutrients, which forces your body out of ketosis stage.

Remember, you need to restart this diet once your body is out of ketosis.

3. Obsessing over weight loss rather than macronutrient intake.

We get it. You are following the Ketogenic diet in order to lose weight, but if you constantly obsess with how much pounds you are shedding, rather than how much macronutrients you need to consume on a daily basis, you may be in for a rude awakening.

In the first few days, you may see little changes in your weight. Some people even gain a few pounds. This is often due to water retention (moisture that your body hoards as it enters the state of ketosis.)
Your body will gradually expel water afterwards when circulatory and gastric systems acclimatize to your dietary changes.

In the meantime, it would be best to keep the weighing scale in the attic or basement.

Direct more of your attention and energy into calculating how much macronutrients you should include in your meals. It is also advisable to constantly update or recalculate as your body adjusts to its dietary changes.

4. Not consuming enough fiber-rich food or drinking higher volumes of water.

Constipation is one of the biggest drawbacks when following the Keto diet. Water is expelled out of the body quickly that this sometimes hinder or delay bowel movement. Instead of using laxatives, try drinking more water and eating food items that are rich in fiber. Both of these can safely be incorporated in your daily meals.

Chapter 4: Ketogenic Diet Safe Food Items and Drinks to Consume

Food items that contain good sources of organic fat and oils are on top of this list. Preferably:

- Omega 3 rich food:
    - American shad
    - Anchovies
    - Beechnuts
    - Beef
    - Broad/fava beans
    - Broccoli
    - Brussels sprouts
    - Cauliflowers
    - Chia seeds
    - Cod liver oil
    - Edamame, soybeans, soy nuts
    - Fish roe
    - Flaxseed, flaxseed oil
    - Halibut
    - Hickory nuts
    - Herring
    - Kale
    - Kidney beans
    - Macadamia nuts
    - Mackerel
    - Navy beans
    - Pecans
    - Pine nuts
    - Pistachios
    - Pumpkin seeds
    - Sardines in brine or oil, bottled or canned
    - Sardines, fresh

- Salmon in brine or oil, bottled or canned
- Salmon, fresh
- Shellfish / seafood
  - Clams
  - Mussels
  - Shrimp or prawns
  - Squids
- Spinach
- Swordfish
- Trout
- Tuna
- Walnuts, walnut oil

- Omega 6 rich food:
  - Almonds
  - Avocado
  - Bacon
  - Beef
  - Black walnuts, black walnut oil
  - Caesar's, French, Honey-Mustard, Italian, and Thousand Island dressings
  - Cheese
    - Cheddar
    - Cream cheese
    - Goat's cheese
    - Gruyere
    - Parmesan
  - Chicken
  - Eggs
  - Ham
  - Mayonnaise
  - Pecan nuts
  - Pine nuts
  - Pork chops, loin, salami, spareribs, ground pork
  - Pumpkin seeds
  - Sesame seeds (not the oil)

- o Squash seeds
- o Sunflower seeds (not the oil)
- o Soybean oil
- o Turkey, turkey bacon, ground turkey
- o Whole milk

- Other sources of good fats/oils:
  - o Animal fats, lard, tallow
  - o Avocado, avocado oil
  - o Butter, clarified butter, ghee
  - o Coconut, coconut oil / palm oil
  - o Eggs
  - o Fatty fish, seafood, roe, fatty fish oil
    - Cod liver oil
  - o Hemp seed oil
  - o Nuts, nut oils
    - Almond, almond oil
    - Cashew, cashew oil
    - Hazelnut, hazelnut oil
    - Macadamia, macadamia oil
    - Walnut, walnut oil
  - o Olive oil

Include moderate amounts of proteins, like:
- Meat
  - o Beef
  - o Goat
  - o Lamb
  - o Pork
  - o Poultry
  - o Veal
- Seafood
  - o Fish
    - Catfish
    - Cod
    - Flounder

- Grouper
- Halibut
- Mackerel
- Salmon
- Snapper
- Trout
- Tuna
- Whitefish
  - Shellfish
    - Clams
    - Crabs
    - Lobsters
    - Mussels
    - Oysters
    - Scallops
    - Shrimps, prawns
    - Squids
    - Scallops
- Whole eggs

Non-starchy, mostly leafy vegetables (and some fruits,) preferably low carbohydrates, and low in Glycemic Index, like:

- Asparagus
- Avocado (fruit)
- Bell peppers (fruit)
- Broccoli
- Carrots
- Cauliflower
- Celery
- Chives
- Coconuts, fresh or dried, not the oil, (fruit)
- Cucumber, (fruit)
- Green beans, snow peas
- Leeks
- Lettuce

- Lemons, limes (fruits)
- Mushrooms
- Onions, shallots, green onions
- Peas
- Spinach
- Squash
- Tomato, (fruit)

Dairy products:

- Cheeses
  - Blue
  - Brie
  - Cheddar
  - Colby jack
  - Cottage cheese
  - Cream cheese
  - Edam
  - Mascarpone
  - Mozzarella
  - Parmesan
  - Ricotta
  - Swiss cheese
- Creams
  - Double cream
  - Half and half
  - Single / table cream
  - Sour cream
  - Whipping cream
- Milks
  - Buttermilk
  - Skim
  - Whole

Nuts and seeds:

- Almonds, almond flour
- Brazil nuts
- Cashew nuts, use sparingly
- Chestnuts
- Chia seeds
- Flax seeds, milled flax seed flour
- Hazelnuts
- Macadamia
- Pine nuts
- Pistachio nuts, use sparingly
- Walnuts

Beverages, all sugar free or sweetened sparingly:
- Coffee, black, with cream
- Herbal infusions
- Tea
- Water

Food Items and Drinks you should Remove or Limit from your Diet

- Breads
- Chocolate and all sugary food items and drinks
- Fruits, most as these have high sugar content. Some berries can be consumed, as long as you use these sparingly
- Margarine
- pasta
- Peanuts
- Vegetable-based oils
  - Canola oil
  - Corn oil
  - Safflower oil
  - Sunflower oil

Chapter 5: 3-Month Meal Plan Sample

This 90-day meal plan is a mere sample. You can/should substitute Keto Diet safe ingredients that are more readily available in your area. Include your favorite food items and drinks as long as these are Ketogenic safe. Always stick to recommended portions per meal to avoid weight gain.

Lastly, do not be afraid to use your favorite Keto-safe ingredients or meals over and over. These would make this diet easier to accept (gastronomically) and prepare, and may save you money in the long run.

Day 1

Breakfast: Coconut - Mango Milkshake
Makes 1 serving
Ingredients:

¼	cup	coconut cream
¾	cup	water
1	cheek, large	mango cheek, ripe or slightly overripe, peeled, roughly chopped
1	Tbsp.	extra virgin coconut oil
1	dab	fresh vanilla scraping (taken from dried vanilla pod, halved, insides scraped)
⅛	tsp.	green stevia, optional

Directions:
1. Combine all ingredients in a blender. Process until smooth. Serve immediately.

Lunch: Anchovy on Avocado Salad
Makes 2 servings, divide into 2 equal portions
Ingredients:

<u>For the salad</u>

4	cups	fresh salad greens of your choice, rinsed, spun-dried, divided into 2 equal portions
1	can, 2 oz. each	anchovy fillets on olive oil, drained well, but reserve some oil for the dressing
2	pieces, large	eggs, hard-boiled, peeled, quartered
1	piece, medium	avocado, just ripe/tender, halved, stone removed, peeled, thinly sliced

<u>For the dressing</u>

1	Tbsp.	lemon juice, freshly squeezed
1	Tbsp.	extra virgin olive oil (from anchovies)
1	tsp.	English or hot mustard
-	dash	sea salt
-	dash	freshly cracked black pepper powder

Directions:
1. <u>For the dressing</u>: Combine all ingredients in a small lidded bottle. Secure lid. Shake well to combine. Set aside.
2. <u>For the salad</u>: Pour dressing on salad greens. Toss well to combine. Divide into 2 equal portions. Place equal portions of salad greens on 2 plates. Dot equal portions of avocadoes, anchovies, and eggs on top. Serve immediately.

Dinner: Minced Beef Stew on Zucchini Noodles
Makes 4 servings, divide into 4 equal portions
Ingredients:

4	pieces, medium	zucchini, processed into long spaghetti-noodles, using a mandolin or spiralizer
4	pieces, large	ripe tomatoes, deseeded, minced
3½	cups	minced beef, 90% lean gluten-free, low-sodium
2	cups	beef broth/stock
1	stalk, large	celery, minced
1	clove, large	garlic, minced
1	piece, large	yellow onion, minced
1	Tbsp.	clarified butter
1	tsp.	olive oil
1	tsp.	dried pepper flakes
-	dash	sea salt, add more if desired
-	dash	freshly cracked black pepper powder

Directions:
1. Pour butter and oil into Dutch oven set over medium heat. Add in celery, garlic and onion. Sauté until limp and transparent. Add in beef, pepper flakes and tomatoes. Stir-fry, breaking up larger clumps of meat as you go.
2. Except for zucchini noodles, add remaining ingredients into Dutch oven. Partially close lid. Let stew cook until broth is reduced by half, about 15 to 20 minutes.
3. To serve: Divide zucchini noodles and stew into 4 equal portions. Place 1 portion of noodles on plate and top off with 1 portion of stew. Serve warm.

Snack: Hard Boiled Egg, large, lightly seasoned, only if needed

Day 2

Breakfast: Blueberry and Cashew Milkshake
Makes 1 serving
Ingredients:

1	cup	cashew milk
¾	cup	frozen blueberries
1	Tbsp.	double cream or whipped cream
1	tsp.	lemon juice, freshly squeezed
⅛	tsp.	green stevia, optional

Directions:
1. Combine all ingredients in a blender. Process until smooth. Serve immediately.

Lunch: Quick-Pickled Mackerel on Open Faced Cucumber Sandwich
Makes 4 servings, divide into 4 equal portions
Ingredients:

For the sandwich

2	pieces, large	cucumbers, halved lengthwise, seeds scooped out, using a vegetable peeler, peel a small section on the unsliced part of the vegetables to form a steady "base," chill well before using
1	head, large	red leaf lettuce, leaves separated, rinsed well, spun-dried, shredded

		chill well before using, divided into 4 equal portions
1	piece, small	lime, quartered, remove pips
2	Tbsp.	apple cider vinegar, divided into 4 (approx. ½ Tbsp. each)

For the mackerel filling

4	pieces, large	Kalamata olives, pitted, minced
4	pieces	cherry or grape tomatoes, quartered, deseeded
1	piece, medium	*jalapeño* pepper, deseeded, minced
1	piece, 6 oz.	mackerel fillet, sliced into thin matchsticks
1	tsp.	clarified butter
1	tsp.	olive oil
1	tsp.	capers in brine, drained well
-	dash	white pepper
-	-	sea salt, only if needed

Directions:

1. <u>For the filling</u>: Pour clarified butter and olive oil into saucepan set over medium heat. Gently fry mackerel pieces until browned. Transfer to plate and cover with aluminum foil.

2. In the same pan, add in tomatoes, capers and olives. Stir-fry until tomatoes are a little wilted. Turn off heat completely before adding in remaining ingredients. Stir. Season according to personal preference.

3. <u>To assemble</u>: Drizzle ½ tablespoon of apple cider vinegar on each cucumber half, cut side up.
4. Place equal amounts of shredded lettuce into cucumber cavities.
5. Add equal portions of warm mackerel on lettuce leaves. This will wilt the vegetables a little. Add in equal portions of tomato-capers mix.
6. Serve cucumber sandwich with lime quarters. Squeeze juice on sandwich prior to eating.

Dinner: Sardine Stuffed Spicy Avocadoes
Makes 4 servings, divide into 4 equal portions
Ingredients:

2	pieces, large	ripe avocado, halved lengthwise, stone removed
1	can, 3.2 oz.	sardines in oil, drained lightly
2	Tbsp.	mayonnaise, commercial blend is fine as long as it is gluten-free, but homemade is better
1	tsp.	dried pepper flakes
1	tsp., heaping	chives, minced, reserve half for garnish
-	dash	sweet paprika powder, add more if desired
-	dash	sea salt, add more if desired
-	dash	turmeric powder, add more if desired
-	dash	white pepper, add more if desired

Directions:
1. Except for avocadoes, combine the rest of the ingredients into a mixing bowl. Whisk well, breaking up larger clumps

of sardines as you go along. Season to taste. Divide into 4
equal portions.

2. Spoon 1 portion into each avocado cavity. Sprinkle chives
    before serving.

Snack: ¼ cup shelled pistachio nuts, lightly seasoned, only if
needed

Day 3

Breakfast: Coconut Mushroom Hash
Makes 4 servings

Ingredients:

20	slices, large	pancetta or bacon, roughly sliced
10	cups	white or button mushrooms, thinly sliced
½	cup	water
2	Tbsp.	wholegrain mustard
1	piece, large	sweet orange, zested, juiced, pips removed
½	cup	thick coconut cream
-	pinch	sea salt
-	pinch	black pepper, add more if desired
-	handful	fresh parsley, roughly chopped, for garnish, optional

Directions:

1. Place pancetta and water in a large non-stick frying pan set over high heat. Let water come to a full boil. This will render fat out of the pancetta. Turn heat to medium setting when pan starts to sizzle. Continue cooking pancetta until most are brown and crisp. With slotted spoon, remove bacon from pan and transfer to a plate.
2. Add in mushrooms into the bacon oil, and cook these until seared on both sides.
3. Except for the bacon, add in remaining ingredients into the pan. Stir and cook until sauce thickens, about 4 to 6

minutes. Season lightly, as the pancetta carries a lot of flavor.

4. <u>To serve</u>: divide mushroom hash and cooked pancetta into 4 equal portions. Place equal portions into individual bowls. Garnish with parsley if using. Serve warm.

Lunch: Stir-Fried Brussels Sprouts with Bacon on Mung Bean Sprout "Noodles"
Makes 4 servings, divide into 4 equal portions

Ingredients:

10	pieces, large	streaky bacon, roughly chopped
½	cup	water
4	cups, heaping	Brussels sprouts, quartered, remove tough ends, but do not remove cores completely
4	cups, heaping	white or button mushrooms, preferably small caps, or approximately the same size as that of the Brussels sprouts, quartered
2	cups	mung bean sprouts, rinsed, drained well, divided into 4 equal portions
1	clove, small	garlic, minced
2	pieces, medium	tomatoes, deseeded, minced
1	piece, medium	white onion, minced
-	-	sea salt, to taste
-	-	white pepper, to taste

Directions:

1. Place bacon and water in a large non-stick frying pan set over high heat. Let water come to a full boil. This will

render fat out of the pancetta. Turn heat to medium setting when pan starts to sizzle. Continue cooking pancetta until most are brown and crisp. With slotted spoon, remove bacon from pan and transfer to a plate.

2. Sauté onions and garlic in bacon oil until limp and aromatic. Add in mushrooms and tomatoes. Cook until mushrooms are fork-tender, about 3 to 5 minutes.

3. Add in Brussels sprouts. Return bacon crisps back into the pan. Stir. Put lid on. Let this cook for 3 minutes, or until Brussels sprouts turn 1 shade lighter. Turn off heat. Season to taste. Divide into 4 equal portions.

4. To assemble: place equal portions of mung bean sprouts on individual plates. Top off with 1 portion of stir-fried vegetables and bacon. Serve warm.

Dinner: Minute Pork Chops with Buttered Shiitake Mushrooms
Makes 4 servings, divide into 4 equal portions
Ingredients:

For the meat

4	pieces, large	boneless pork chops, rinds removed, using a meat mallet, pound the chops into ½ inch thick or thinner
-	dash	sea salt
-	dash	black pepper
1	tsp.	clarified butter
1	tsp.	olive oil

For the mushrooms

4	cups	dried shiitake mushrooms, soaked in water for at least 3 hours, stems discarded, caps julienned, reserve...
½	cup	soaking liquid
2	cups	mushroom or vegetable broth/stock, gluten-free, low-sodium
-	-	olive oil, if needed
1	tsp.	butter

Directions:
1. <u>For pork chops</u>: Season meat with salt and pepper. Pour oil and butter into non-stick frying pan set over medium heat.
2. Fry pork chops one at a time until golden brown on both sides. Transfer cooked meat on plate. Place a sheet of aluminum foil on top. Let meat rest while you cook mushrooms.
3. <u>For the mushrooms</u>: In the same pan, stir fry mushrooms in small batches for 3 to 5 minutes, adding oil as needed.

This will impart a smoky flavor. Place partially cooked mushrooms in a bowl, while you continue cooking the rest.

4. Return mushrooms into frying pan. Except for butter, pour in remaining ingredients into pan. Stir. Put lid on. Let mushrooms stew until fork tender, and liquid is reduced in half. Turn off heat. Add butter prior to assembling dish. Divide into 4 equal portions.

5. <u>To assemble</u>: Place 1 pork chop on a plate. Top with 1 portion of buttery mushrooms. Serve warm.

Snack: ¼ cup fried green peas, lightly salted, only if needed

Day 4

Breakfast: Almond - Strawberry Milkshake
Makes 1 serving
Ingredients:

1	cup	almond milk
½	cup	frozen strawberries
1	Tbsp.	double or whipped cream
1	pinch	nutmeg powder
⅛	tsp.	green stevia, optional

Directions:

1. Combine all ingredients in a blender. Process until smooth. Serve immediately.

Lunch: Cucumber and Tuna Salad
Makes 2 servings, divide into 2 equal portions
Ingredients:

For the salad

4	cups	fresh salad greens of your choice, rinsed, spun-dried, divided into 2 equal portions
2	pieces, 3 oz. each	tuna fillets, diced into bite-sized pieces
2	pieces, large	eggs, hard-boiled, peeled, quartered
2	pieces, large	cucumbers, halved, deseeded, diced into bite-sized pieces
1	tsp.	extra virgin olive oil
-	dash	sea salt
-	dash	freshly cracked black pepper powder

For the dressing

1	Tbsp.	apple cider vinegar

1	Tbsp.	extra virgin olive oil
1	tsp.	English or hot mustard

Directions:

1. <u>For the dressing</u>: Combine all ingredients in a small lidded bottle. Secure lid. Shake well to combine. Set aside.
2. <u>For the salad</u>: Pour oil into non-stick frying pan set over medium heat. Lightly season tuna cubes with salt and pepper. Sear tuna cubes until just golden. Transfer cubes to a plate, and place a sheet of aluminum foil on top.
3. <u>P</u>our dressing on salad greens. Toss well to combine. Divide into 2 equal portions. Place equal portions of salad greens on 2 plates. Dot equal portions of cucumbers, cooked tuna cubes and eggs on top. Serve immediately.

Dinner: Minced Beef Stew on Zucchini Noodles
See Day 1 for Recipe
Snack: Hard Boiled Egg, large, lightly seasoned, only if needed

Day 5

Breakfast: Creamy Blueberries in Cream Cheese Flapjacks with Bacon
Makes 1 serving
Ingredients:

2	oz.	cream cheese, at room temperature, approx. ¼ cup
2	pieces, large	eggs
1	pinch	cinnamon powder
1	pinch	nutmeg powder
⅛	tsp.	green stevia, optional
-	-	coconut oil, for greasing
<u>For garnish</u>		
½	cup	frozen blueberries, thawed, substitute any seasonal or local berries available, divided
4	strips	cooked bacon, halved

Directions:

1. Except for garnishes and oil, whisk ingredients together until smooth.
2. In frying pan set over medium heat, pour just enough oil to grease cooking surface lightly.
3. Pour half of batter mix into frying pan. Cook until edges are set and center is still liquid. Add half portion of blueberries in center.
4. Carefully flip flapjack and cook other side. Transfer to a plate. Repeat step for other half of batter.
5. To assemble: stack flapjacks on a plate. Serve with crispy bacon on the side.

Lunch: Spicy Sausage Salad with Asparagus
Makes 4 servings, divide into 4 equal portions
Ingredients:

For the salad

1	tsp.	olive oil, for searing
1	link	Bratwurst sausage, thickly sliced
1	link	Hungarian sausage, thickly sliced
1	link	Kielbasa sausage, thickly sliced
1	link	*Schublig* sausage, thickly sliced
½	cup	apple cider vinegar
1	Tbsp.	balsamic vinegar
1	piece, large	onion, julienned
1	piece, large	green chili, cored, deseeded, julienned
1	piece, small	bell pepper, cored, deseeded, julienned

For garnish

| 4 | handfuls, generous | asparagus spears, thick, blanched/steamed |
| 1 | handful, generous | fresh parsley, roughly chopped, optional |

Directions:
1. Pour oil into large non-stick frying pan set over high heat. Fry sausages in batches, searing cut sides until golden. Transfer cooked pieces onto a plate. Repeat step until all sausages are cooked.
2. Return sausages into frying pan. Add in remaining ingredients and toss well to combine. Turn off heat. Divide into 4 equal portions.
3. To assemble: place 1 portion of cooked asparagus spears on a plate. Make crisscross or overlaying patterns, if desired.
4. Top off with 1 portion of sausage salad. Garnish with fresh parsley, if using. Serve warm.

Dinner: Beefy and Spicy Chili
Makes 8 servings, divide into 8 equal portions
Ingredients:

8	strips, thick	uncooked bacon, roughly chopped
¼	cup	water
2	Tbsp.	butter
1	Tbsp.	white vinegar
1	can, 16 oz.	diced tomatoes
1	can, 15/16 oz.	white beans, rinsed, drained well
1	pound	ground beef, 80% lean
1	tsp.	dried pepper flakes
1	tsp.	coriander powder
1	tsp.	cumin powder
1	tsp.	oregano powder
1	clove, small	garlic, minced

1	piece, large	onion, minced
1	piece, small	bird's eye chili, minced (remove seeds if you want less spice)
-	-	sea salt and white pepper, to taste
¾	cup	cream cheese, at room temperature
½	tsp., each portion	sour cream, at room temperature

Directions:

1. Pour water and uncooked bacon into large Dutch oven set over high heat. Let fat render out, and cook bacon until lightly crisp. Remove bacon to a plate.
2. Add in garlic and onion. Cook until limp and transparent. Add in ground beef and cook until browned, breaking up larger clumps of mea as you go.
3. Except for sour cream and cream cheese, add in remaining ingredients. Stir. Season lightly. Put lid on. Wait for chili to boil. Turn down heat to lowest setting.
4. Let chili simmer for 20 to 30 minutes, stirring once in a while just to make sure nothing sticks to bottom of pan.
5. Turn off heat. Pour in cream cheese. Stir. Let chili cool slightly.
6. To assemble: divide stew into 8 equal portions. Ladle 1 portion into individual bowl. Top off with ½ teaspoon sour cream. Serve warm.

Snack: ¼ cup garlic-roasted almonds or cashew nuts, only if needed

Day 6

Breakfast: Blueberry and Cashew Milkshake
See Day 2 for Recipe

Lunch: Quick-Pickled Mackerel on Open Faced Cucumber
Sandwich
See Day 2 for Recipe

Dinner: Sardine Stuffed Spicy Avocadoes
See Day 2 for Recipe

Snack: ¼ cup shelled pistachio nuts, lightly seasoned, only if
needed

Day 7

Breakfast: Coconut Mushroom Hash
See Day 3 for Recipes

Lunch: Stir-Fried Brussels Sprouts with Bacon on Mung Bean
Sprout "Noodles"
See Day 3 for Recipes

Dinner: Minute Pork Chops with Buttered Shiitake Mushrooms
See Day 3 for Recipes

Snack: ¼ cup fried green peas, lightly salted, only if needed

Day 8

Breakfast: Creamy Cream Cheese Flapjacks with Ham and Chives
Makes 1 serving
Ingredients:

4	stalks	chives, roots removed, rinsed well, minced
2	oz.	cream cheese, at room temperature, approx. ¼ cup
2	pieces, large	eggs
2	slices, thick	cooked ham, diced, divided, add more if desired
-	dash	sea salt
-	dash	white pepper
-	-	coconut oil, for greasing

Directions:
1. Except for oil, whisk ingredients together until smooth.
2. In a frying pan set over medium heat, pour just enough oil to lightly grease cooking surface.
3. Pour half of batter mix into frying pan. Cook until edges are set and center is still liquid. Add half portion of diced ham in center.
4. Carefully flip flapjack and cook other side. Transfer to a plate. Repeat step for other half of batter.
5. To assemble: stack flapjacks on a plate. Serve warm.

Lunch: Avocado and Tuna _Ceviche_ on _Jicama_ Slices
Makes 6 servings, divide into 6 equal portions
Ingredients:

2	pieces, medium	fresh _jicama_, peeled, sliced into 6 thick, equal sized medallions, this

will serve as base of salad, mince leftover *jicama* pieces for *ceviche*

<u>For *ceviche*</u>

1	pound	fresh tuna fillet, diced into bite-sized pieces, refrigerate until ready to use
1	piece, medium	ripe avocado, stone removed, peeled, diced into bite-sized pieces
1	piece, small	shallot, minced
1	piece, small	green chili, deseeded, minced
1	clove, small	garlic, minced
1	Tbsp.	capers in brine/oil, drained well
1	Tbsp.	apple cider vinegar
-	-	sea salt, to taste
-	-	black pepper, to taste
½	cup	lemon juice, freshly squeezed
¼	cup	extra virgin olive oil
1	handful, generous	fresh cilantro, minced, for garnish, optional

Directions:

1. In a small bowl, add shallots and a large pinch of salt. Set aside for at least 30 minutes. Rinse shallots well under running water. Squeeze out excess moisture. Drain well.
2. Place shallot into large mixing bowl. Combine with apple cider vinegar, black pepper, capers, garlic, green chili, lemon juice, olive oil. Mix gently so as not to crush capers.
3. Add in avocadoes, *jicama,* and tuna when you are ready to serve. Toss gently to combine. Divide into 6 equal portions.

4. <u>To assemble</u>: spoon 1 portion of *ceviche* on chilled *jicama* slice, but leave out as much liquid as possible. Serve immediately.

Dinner: Pork Tenderloin Stir-Fry with Cashew Nuts on Zucchini Noodles
Makes 4 servings, divide into 4 equal portions
Ingredients:

1	pound	pork tenderloin, trimmed well, membranes removed, julienned
1	piece, medium	white onion, julienned
1	piece, medium	red bell pepper, julienned
1	piece, small	green chili, deseeded, julienned
-	-	sea salt and white pepper, to taste
1	tsp.	clarified butter
½	tsp.	olive oil
1	cup	garlic-roasted cashew nuts
1	piece, large	zucchini, processed into flat, ribbon like noodles using a vegetable peeler or spiralizer, divide into 4 equal portions, add more if desired

Directions:

1. Place equal portions of zucchini noodles into individual plates. Set aside.
2. Lightly season pork tenderloin with sea salt and white pepper.
3. Pour oil and butter into large non-stick frying pan set over medium heat.
4. Fry pork tenderloin strips in batches, until golden brown. Transfer cooked meat onto plates. Place a sheet of aluminum foil on top. Repeat step until all meat is cooked.
5. In the same pan, sauté bell pepper, onion and chili until onions turn transparent. Season with a little salt.
6. Return pork tenderloin to the pan. Stir. Cook for another minute. Turn off heat. Divide into 4 equal portions.
7. Ladle these immediately on the zucchini noodles. Top off with equal portions of garlic-roasted cashew nuts. Serve immediately.

Snack: ½ cup fresh berries of choice, only if needed

Day 9

Breakfast: Coconut - Mango Milkshake
See Day 1 for recipe

Lunch: Anchovy on Avocado Salad
See Day 1 for recipe

Dinner: Minced Beef Stew on Zucchini Noodles
See Day 1 for recipe

Snack: Hard Boiled Egg, large, lightly seasoned, only if needed

Day 10

Breakfast: Creamy Blueberries in Cream Cheese Flapjacks with Bacon
See Day 5 for Recipe

Lunch: Spicy Sausage Salad with Asparagus
See Day 5 for Recipe

Dinner: Beefy and Spicy Chili
See Day 5 for Recipe

Snack: ¼ cup garlic-roasted almonds or cashew nuts, only if needed

Day 11

Breakfast: Blueberry and Cashew Milkshake
See Day 2 for Recipe

Lunch: Quick-Pickled Mackerel on Open Faced Cucumber
Sandwich
See Day 2 for Recipe

Dinner: Sardine Stuffed Spicy Avocadoes
See Day 2 for Recipe

Snack: ¼ cup shelled pistachio nuts, lightly seasoned, only if
needed

Day 12

Breakfast: Coconut Mushroom Hash
See Day 3 for Recipes

Lunch: Stir-Fried Brussels Sprouts with Bacon on Mung Bean
Sprout "Noodles"
See Day 3 for Recipes

Dinner: Minute Pork Chops with Buttered Shiitake Mushrooms
See Day 3 for Recipes

Snack: ¼ cup fried green peas, lightly salted, only if needed

Day 13

Breakfast: Creamy Blueberries in Cream Cheese Flapjacks with Bacon
See Day 5 for Recipe

Lunch: Spicy Sausage Salad with Asparagus
See Day 5 for Recipe

Dinner: Beefy and Spicy Chili
See Day 5 for Recipe

Snack: ¼ cup garlic-roasted almonds or cashew nuts, only if needed

Day 14

Breakfast: Creamy Cream Cheese Flapjacks with Ham and Chives
See Day 8 for Recipe

Lunch: Avocado and Tuna *Ceviche* on *Jicama* Slices
See Day 8 for Recipe

Dinner: Pork Tenderloin Stir-Fry with Cashew Nuts on Zucchini Noodles
See Day 8 for Recipe

Snack: ½ cup fresh berries of choice, only if needed

Day 15

Breakfast: Almond - Strawberry Milkshake
See Day 4 for recipe

Lunch: Cucumber and Tuna Salad
See Day 4 for recipe

Dinner: Minced Beef Stew on Zucchini Noodles
See Day 1 for recipe

Snack: Hard Boiled Egg, large, lightly seasoned, only if needed

Day 16

Breakfast: Coconut Mushroom Hash
See Day 3 for Recipes

Lunch: Stir-Fried Brussels Sprouts with Bacon on Mung Bean Sprout "Noodles"
See Day 3 for Recipes

Dinner: Minute Pork Chops with Buttered Shiitake Mushrooms
See Day 3 for Recipes

Snack: ¼ cup fried green peas, lightly salted, only if needed

Day 17

Breakfast: Blueberry and Cashew Milkshake
See Day 2 for Recipe

Lunch: Quick-Pickled Mackerel on Open Faced Cucumber
Sandwich
See Day 2 for Recipe

Dinner: Sardine Stuffed Spicy Avocadoes
See Day 2 for Recipe

Snack: ¼ cup shelled pistachio nuts, lightly seasoned, only if
needed

Day 18

Breakfast: Creamy Blueberries in Cream Cheese Flapjacks with
Bacon
See Day 5 for Recipe

Lunch: Spicy Sausage Salad with Asparagus
See Day 5 for Recipe

Dinner: Beefy and Spicy Chili
See Day 5 for Recipe

Snack: ¼ cup garlic-roasted almonds or cashew nuts, only if
needed

Day 19

Breakfast: Coconut - Mango Milkshake
See Day 1 for recipe

Lunch: Anchovy on Avocado Salad
See Day 1 for recipe

Dinner: Minced Beef Stew on Zucchini Noodles
See Day 1 for recipe

Snack: Hard Boiled Egg, large, lightly seasoned, only if needed

Day 20

Breakfast: Blueberry and Cashew Milkshake
See Day 2 for Recipe

Lunch: Quick-Pickled Mackerel on Open Faced Cucumber
Sandwich
See Day 2 for Recipe

Dinner: Sardine Stuffed Spicy Avocadoes
See Day 2 for Recipe

Snack: ¼ cup shelled pistachio nuts, lightly seasoned, only if
needed

Day 21

Breakfast: Coconut Mushroom Hash
See Day 3 for Recipes

Lunch: Stir-Fried Brussels Sprouts with Bacon on Mung Bean Sprout "Noodles"
See Day 3 for Recipes

Dinner: Minute Pork Chops with Buttered Shiitake Mushrooms
See Day 3 for Recipes

Snack: ¼ cup fried green peas, lightly salted, only if needed

Day 22

Breakfast: Creamy Blueberries in Cream Cheese Flapjacks with Bacon
See Day 5 for Recipe

Lunch: Spicy Sausage Salad with Asparagus
See Day 5 for Recipe

Dinner: Beefy and Spicy Chili
See Day 5 for Recipe

Snack: ¼ cup garlic-roasted almonds or cashew nuts, only if needed

Day 23

Breakfast: Creamy Cream Cheese Flapjacks with Ham and Chives
See Day 8 for Recipe

Lunch: Avocado and Tuna *Ceviche* on *Jicama* Slices
See Day 8 for Recipe

Dinner: Pork Tenderloin Stir-Fry with Cashew Nuts on Zucchini Noodles
See Day 8 for Recipe

Snack: ½ cup fresh berries of choice, only if needed

Day 24

Breakfast: Coconut Mushroom Hash
See Day 3 for Recipes

Lunch: Stir-Fried Brussels Sprouts with Bacon on Mung Bean Sprout "Noodles"
See Day 3 for Recipes

Dinner: Minute Pork Chops with Buttered Shiitake Mushrooms
See Day 3 for Recipes

Snack: ¼ cup fried green peas, lightly salted, only if needed

Day 25

Breakfast: Almond - Strawberry Milkshake
See Day 4 for recipe

Lunch: Cucumber and Tuna Salad
See Day 4 for recipe

Dinner: Minced Beef Stew on Zucchini Noodles
See Day 1 for recipe

Snack: Hard Boiled Egg, large, lightly seasoned, only if needed

Day 26

Breakfast: Creamy Blueberries in Cream Cheese Flapjacks with Bacon
See Day 5 for Recipe

Lunch: Spicy Sausage Salad with Asparagus
See Day 5 for Recipe

Dinner: Beefy and Spicy Chili
See Day 5 for Recipe

Snack: ¼ cup garlic-roasted almonds or cashew nuts, only if needed

Day 27

Breakfast: Creamy Cream Cheese Flapjacks with Ham and Chives
See Day 8 for Recipe

Lunch: Avocado and Tuna *Ceviche* on *Jicama* Slices
See Day 8 for Recipe

Dinner: Pork Tenderloin Stir-Fry with Cashew Nuts on Zucchini Noodles
See Day 8 for Recipe

Snack: ½ cup fresh berries of choice, only if needed

Day 28

Breakfast: Coconut Mushroom Hash
See Day 3 for Recipes

Lunch: Stir-Fried Brussels Sprouts with Bacon on Mung Bean Sprout "Noodles"
See Day 3 for Recipes

Dinner: Minute Pork Chops with Buttered Shiitake Mushrooms
See Day 3 for Recipes

Snack: ¼ cup fried green peas, lightly salted, only if needed

Day 29

Breakfast: Blueberry and Cashew Milkshake
See Day 2 for Recipe

Lunch: Quick-Pickled Mackerel on Open Faced Cucumber
Sandwich
See Day 2 for Recipe

Dinner: Sardine Stuffed Spicy Avocadoes
See Day 2 for Recipe

Snack: ¼ cup shelled pistachio nuts, lightly seasoned, only if
needed

Day 30

Breakfast: Blueberry and Cashew Milkshake
See Day 2 for Recipe

Lunch: Quick-Pickled Mackerel on Open Faced Cucumber
Sandwich
See Day 2 for Recipe

Dinner: Sardine Stuffed Spicy Avocadoes
See Day 2 for Recipe

Snack: ¼ cup shelled pistachio nuts, lightly seasoned, only if
needed

Day 31

Breakfast: Creamy Blueberries in Cream Cheese Flapjacks with Bacon
See Day 5 for Recipe

Lunch: Spicy Sausage Salad with Asparagus
See Day 5 for Recipe

Dinner: Beefy and Spicy Chili
See Day 5 for Recipe

Snack: ¼ cup garlic-roasted almonds or cashew nuts, only if needed

Day 32

Breakfast: Creamy Cream Cheese Flapjacks with Ham and Chives
See Day 8 for Recipe

Lunch: Avocado and Tuna _Ceviche_ on _Jicama_ Slices
See Day 8 for Recipe

Dinner: Pork Tenderloin Stir-Fry with Cashew Nuts on Zucchini Noodles
See Day 8 for Recipe

Snack: ½ cup fresh berries of choice, only if needed

Day 33

Breakfast: Coconut - Mango Milkshake
See Day 1 for recipe

Lunch: Anchovy on Avocado Salad
See Day 1 for recipe

Dinner: Minced Beef Stew on Zucchini Noodles
See Day 1 for recipe

Snack: Hard Boiled Egg, large, lightly seasoned, only if needed

Day 34

Breakfast: Blueberry and Cashew Milkshake
See Day 2 for Recipe

Lunch: Quick-Pickled Mackerel on Open Faced Cucumber Sandwich
See Day 2 for Recipe

Dinner: Sardine Stuffed Spicy Avocadoes
See Day 2 for Recipe

Snack: ¼ cup shelled pistachio nuts, lightly seasoned, only if needed

Day 35

Breakfast: Coconut Mushroom Hash
See Day 3 for Recipes

Lunch: Stir-Fried Brussels Sprouts with Bacon on Mung Bean Sprout "Noodles"
See Day 3 for Recipes

Dinner: Minute Pork Chops with Buttered Shiitake Mushrooms
See Day 3 for Recipes

Snack: ¼ cup fried green peas, lightly salted, only if needed

Day 36

Breakfast: Creamy Blueberries in Cream Cheese Flapjacks with Bacon
See Day 5 for Recipe

Lunch: Spicy Sausage Salad with Asparagus
See Day 5 for Recipe

Dinner: Beefy and Spicy Chili
See Day 5 for Recipe

Snack: ¼ cup garlic-roasted almonds or cashew nuts, only if needed

Day 37

Breakfast: Almond - Strawberry Milkshake
See Day 4 for recipe

Lunch: Cucumber and Tuna Salad
See Day 4 for recipe

Dinner: Minced Beef Stew on Zucchini Noodles
See Day 1 for recipe

Snack: Hard Boiled Egg, large, lightly seasoned, only if needed

Day 38

Breakfast: Creamy Cream Cheese Flapjacks with Ham and Chives
See Day 8 for Recipe

Lunch: Avocado and Tuna *Ceviche* on *Jicama* Slices
See Day 8 for Recipe

Dinner: Pork Tenderloin Stir-Fry with Cashew Nuts on Zucchini Noodles
See Day 8 for Recipe

Snack: ½ cup fresh berries of choice, only if needed

Day 39

Breakfast: Blueberry and Cashew Milkshake
See Day 2 for Recipe

Lunch: Quick-Pickled Mackerel on Open Faced Cucumber Sandwich
See Day 2 for Recipe

Dinner: Sardine Stuffed Spicy Avocadoes
See Day 2 for Recipe

Snack: ¼ cup shelled pistachio nuts, lightly seasoned, only if needed

Day 40

Breakfast: Creamy Blueberries in Cream Cheese Flapjacks with Bacon
See Day 5 for Recipe

Lunch: Spicy Sausage Salad with Asparagus
See Day 5 for Recipe

Dinner: Beefy and Spicy Chili
See Day 5 for Recipe

Snack: ¼ cup garlic-roasted almonds or cashew nuts, only if needed

Day 41

Breakfast: Coconut Mushroom Hash
See Day 3 for Recipes

Lunch: Stir-Fried Brussels Sprouts with Bacon on Mung Bean Sprout "Noodles"
See Day 3 for Recipes

Dinner: Minute Pork Chops with Buttered Shiitake Mushrooms
See Day 3 for Recipes

Snack: ¼ cup fried green peas, lightly salted, only if needed

Day 42

Breakfast: Coconut - Mango Milkshake
See Day 1 for recipe

Lunch: Anchovy on Avocado Salad
See Day 1 for recipe

Dinner: Minced Beef Stew on Zucchini Noodles
See Day 1 for recipe

Snack: Hard Boiled Egg, large, lightly seasoned, only if needed

Day 43

Breakfast: Blueberry and Cashew Milkshake
See Day 2 for Recipe

Lunch: Quick-Pickled Mackerel on Open Faced Cucumber
Sandwich
See Day 2 for Recipe

Dinner: Sardine Stuffed Spicy Avocadoes
See Day 2 for Recipe

Snack: ¼ cup shelled pistachio nuts, lightly seasoned, only if
needed

Day 44

Breakfast: Coconut Mushroom Hash
See Day 3 for Recipes

Lunch: Stir-Fried Brussels Sprouts with Bacon on Mung Bean
Sprout "Noodles"
See Day 3 for Recipes

Dinner: Minute Pork Chops with Buttered Shiitake Mushrooms
See Day 3 for Recipes

Snack: ¼ cup fried green peas, lightly salted, only if needed

Day 45

Breakfast: Creamy Blueberries in Cream Cheese Flapjacks with Bacon
See Day 5 for Recipe

Lunch: Spicy Sausage Salad with Asparagus
See Day 5 for Recipe

Dinner: Beefy and Spicy Chili
See Day 5 for Recipe

Snack: ¼ cup garlic-roasted almonds or cashew nuts, only if needed

Day 46

Breakfast: Creamy Cream Cheese Flapjacks with Ham and Chives
See Day 8 for Recipe

Lunch: Avocado and Tuna *Ceviche* on *Jicama* Slices
See Day 8 for Recipe

Dinner: Pork Tenderloin Stir-Fry with Cashew Nuts on Zucchini Noodles
See Day 8 for Recipe

Snack: ½ cup fresh berries of choice, only if needed

Day 47

Breakfast: Coconut Mushroom Hash
See Day 3 for Recipes

Lunch: Stir-Fried Brussels Sprouts with Bacon on Mung Bean Sprout "Noodles"
See Day 3 for Recipes

Dinner: Minute Pork Chops with Buttered Shiitake Mushrooms
See Day 3 for Recipes

Snack: ¼ cup fried green peas, lightly salted, only if needed

Day 48

Breakfast: Creamy Blueberries in Cream Cheese Flapjacks with Bacon
See Day 5 for Recipe

Lunch: Spicy Sausage Salad with Asparagus
See Day 5 for Recipe

Dinner: Beefy and Spicy Chili
See Day 5 for Recipe

Snack: ¼ cup garlic-roasted almonds or cashew nuts, only if needed

Day 49

Breakfast: Almond - Strawberry Milkshake
See Day 4 for recipe

Lunch: Cucumber and Tuna Salad
See Day 4 for recipe

Dinner: Minced Beef Stew on Zucchini Noodles
See Day 1 for recipe

Snack: Hard Boiled Egg, large, lightly seasoned, only if needed

Day 50

Breakfast: Blueberry and Cashew Milkshake
See Day 2 for Recipe

Lunch: Quick-Pickled Mackerel on Open Faced Cucumber
Sandwich
See Day 2 for Recipe

Dinner: Sardine Stuffed Spicy Avocadoes
See Day 2 for Recipe

Snack: ¼ cup shelled pistachio nuts, lightly seasoned, only if
needed

Day 51

Breakfast: Coconut Mushroom Hash
See Day 3 for Recipes

Lunch: Stir-Fried Brussels Sprouts with Bacon on Mung Bean Sprout "Noodles"
See Day 3 for Recipes

Dinner: Minute Pork Chops with Buttered Shiitake Mushrooms
See Day 3 for Recipes

Snack: ¼ cup fried green peas, lightly salted, only if needed

Day 52

Breakfast: Creamy Blueberries in Cream Cheese Flapjacks with Bacon
See Day 5 for Recipe

Lunch: Spicy Sausage Salad with Asparagus
See Day 5 for Recipe

Dinner: Beefy and Spicy Chili
See Day 5 for Recipe

Snack: ¼ cup garlic-roasted almonds or cashew nuts, only if needed

Day 53

Breakfast: Creamy Cream Cheese Flapjacks with Ham and Chives
See Day 8 for Recipe

Lunch: Avocado and Tuna *Ceviche* on *Jicama* Slices
See Day 8 for Recipe

Dinner: Pork Tenderloin Stir-Fry with Cashew Nuts on Zucchini Noodles
See Day 8 for Recipe

Snack: ½ cup fresh berries of choice, only if needed

Day 54

Breakfast: Coconut Mushroom Hash
See Day 3 for Recipes

Lunch: Stir-Fried Brussels Sprouts with Bacon on Mung Bean Sprout "Noodles"
See Day 3 for Recipes

Dinner: Minute Pork Chops with Buttered Shiitake Mushrooms
See Day 3 for Recipes

Snack: ¼ cup fried green peas, lightly salted, only if needed

Day 55

Breakfast: Coconut - Mango Milkshake
See Day 1 for recipe

Lunch: Anchovy on Avocado Salad
See Day 1 for recipe

Dinner: Minced Beef Stew on Zucchini Noodles
See Day 1 for recipe

Snack: Hard Boiled Egg, large, lightly seasoned, only if needed

Day 56

Breakfast: Blueberry and Cashew Milkshake
See Day 2 for Recipe

Lunch: Quick-Pickled Mackerel on Open Faced Cucumber
Sandwich
See Day 2 for Recipe

Dinner: Sardine Stuffed Spicy Avocadoes
See Day 2 for Recipe

Snack: ¼ cup shelled pistachio nuts, lightly seasoned, only if
needed

Day 57

Breakfast: Creamy Blueberries in Cream Cheese Flapjacks with Bacon
See Day 5 for Recipe

Lunch: Spicy Sausage Salad with Asparagus
See Day 5 for Recipe

Dinner: Beefy and Spicy Chili
See Day 5 for Recipe

Snack: ¼ cup garlic-roasted almonds or cashew nuts, only if needed

Day 58

Breakfast: Coconut Mushroom Hash
See Day 3 for Recipes

Lunch: Stir-Fried Brussels Sprouts with Bacon on Mung Bean Sprout "Noodles"
See Day 3 for Recipes

Dinner: Minute Pork Chops with Buttered Shiitake Mushrooms
See Day 3 for Recipes

Snack: ¼ cup fried green peas, lightly salted, only if needed

Day 59

Breakfast: Blueberry and Cashew Milkshake
See Day 2 for Recipe

Lunch: Quick-Pickled Mackerel on Open Faced Cucumber
Sandwich
See Day 2 for Recipe

Dinner: Sardine Stuffed Spicy Avocadoes
See Day 2 for Recipe

Snack: ¼ cup shelled pistachio nuts, lightly seasoned, only if
needed

Day 60

Breakfast: Almond - Strawberry Milkshake
See Day 4 for recipe

Lunch: Cucumber and Tuna Salad
See Day 4 for recipe

Dinner: Minced Beef Stew on Zucchini Noodles
See Day 1 for recipe

Snack: Hard Boiled Egg, large, lightly seasoned, only if needed

Day 61

Breakfast: Creamy Blueberries in Cream Cheese Flapjacks with Bacon
See Day 5 for Recipe

Lunch: Spicy Sausage Salad with Asparagus
See Day 5 for Recipe

Dinner: Beefy and Spicy Chili
See Day 5 for Recipe

Snack: ¼ cup garlic-roasted almonds or cashew nuts, only if needed

Day 62

Breakfast: Creamy Cream Cheese Flapjacks with Ham and Chives
See Day 8 for Recipe

Lunch: Avocado and Tuna *Ceviche* on *Jicama* Slices
See Day 8 for Recipe

Dinner: Pork Tenderloin Stir-Fry with Cashew Nuts on Zucchini Noodles
See Day 8 for Recipe

Snack: ½ cup fresh berries of choice, only if needed

Day 63

Breakfast: Coconut Mushroom Hash
See Day 3 for Recipes

Lunch: Stir-Fried Brussels Sprouts with Bacon on Mung Bean Sprout "Noodles"
See Day 3 for Recipes

Dinner: Minute Pork Chops with Buttered Shiitake Mushrooms
See Day 3 for Recipes

Snack: ¼ cup fried green peas, lightly salted, only if needed

Day 64

Breakfast: Coconut - Mango Milkshake
See Day 1 for recipe

Lunch: Anchovy on Avocado Salad
See Day 1 for recipe

Dinner: Minced Beef Stew on Zucchini Noodles
See Day 1 for recipe

Snack: Hard Boiled Egg, large, lightly seasoned, only if needed

Day 65

Breakfast: Blueberry and Cashew Milkshake
See Day 2 for Recipe

Lunch: Quick-Pickled Mackerel on Open Faced Cucumber Sandwich
See Day 2 for Recipe

Dinner: Sardine Stuffed Spicy Avocadoes
See Day 2 for Recipe

Snack: ¼ cup shelled pistachio nuts, lightly seasoned, only if needed

Day 66

Breakfast: Coconut Mushroom Hash
See Day 3 for Recipes

Lunch: Stir-Fried Brussels Sprouts with Bacon on Mung Bean Sprout "Noodles"
See Day 3 for Recipes

Dinner: Minute Pork Chops with Buttered Shiitake Mushrooms
See Day 3 for Recipes

Snack: ¼ cup fried green peas, lightly salted, only if needed

Day 67

Breakfast: Creamy Blueberries in Cream Cheese Flapjacks with Bacon
See Day 5 for Recipe

Lunch: Spicy Sausage Salad with Asparagus
See Day 5 for Recipe

Dinner: Beefy and Spicy Chili
See Day 5 for Recipe

Snack: ¼ cup garlic-roasted almonds or cashew nuts, only if needed

Day 68

Breakfast: Almond - Strawberry Milkshake
See Day 4 for recipe

Lunch: Cucumber and Tuna Salad
See Day 4 for recipe

Dinner: Minced Beef Stew on Zucchini Noodles
See Day 1 for recipe

Snack: Hard Boiled Egg, large, lightly seasoned, only if needed

Day 69

Breakfast: Creamy Cream Cheese Flapjacks with Ham and Chives
See Day 8 for Recipe

Lunch: Avocado and Tuna *Ceviche* on *Jicama* Slices
See Day 8 for Recipe

Dinner: Pork Tenderloin Stir-Fry with Cashew Nuts on Zucchini Noodles
See Day 8 for Recipe

Snack: ½ cup fresh berries of choice, only if needed

Day 70

Breakfast: Blueberry and Cashew Milkshake
See Day 2 for Recipe

Lunch: Quick-Pickled Mackerel on Open Faced Cucumber Sandwich
See Day 2 for Recipe

Dinner: Sardine Stuffed Spicy Avocadoes
See Day 2 for Recipe

Snack: ¼ cup shelled pistachio nuts, lightly seasoned, only if needed

Day 71

Breakfast: Coconut Mushroom Hash
See Day 3 for Recipes

Lunch: Stir-Fried Brussels Sprouts with Bacon on Mung Bean
Sprout "Noodles"
See Day 3 for Recipes

Dinner: Minute Pork Chops with Buttered Shiitake Mushrooms
See Day 3 for Recipes

Snack: ¼ cup fried green peas, lightly salted, only if needed

Day 72

Breakfast: Creamy Blueberries in Cream Cheese Flapjacks with
Bacon
See Day 5 for Recipe

Lunch: Spicy Sausage Salad with Asparagus
See Day 5 for Recipe

Dinner: Beefy and Spicy Chili
See Day 5 for Recipe

Snack: ¼ cup garlic-roasted almonds or cashew nuts, only if
needed

Day 73

Breakfast: Coconut - Mango Milkshake
See Day 1 for recipe

Lunch: Anchovy on Avocado Salad
See Day 1 for recipe

Dinner: Minced Beef Stew on Zucchini Noodles
See Day 1 for recipe

Snack: Hard Boiled Egg, large, lightly seasoned, only if needed

Day 74

Breakfast: Blueberry and Cashew Milkshake
See Day 2 for Recipe

Lunch: Quick-Pickled Mackerel on Open Faced Cucumber
Sandwich
See Day 2 for Recipe

Dinner: Sardine Stuffed Spicy Avocadoes
See Day 2 for Recipe

Snack: ¼ cup shelled pistachio nuts, lightly seasoned, only if
needed

Day 75

Breakfast: Coconut Mushroom Hash
See Day 3 for Recipes

Lunch: Stir-Fried Brussels Sprouts with Bacon on Mung Bean Sprout "Noodles"
See Day 3 for Recipes

Dinner: Minute Pork Chops with Buttered Shiitake Mushrooms
See Day 3 for Recipes

Snack: ¼ cup fried green peas, lightly salted, only if needed

Day 76

Breakfast: Creamy Blueberries in Cream Cheese Flapjacks with Bacon
See Day 5 for Recipe

Lunch: Spicy Sausage Salad with Asparagus
See Day 5 for Recipe

Dinner: Beefy and Spicy Chili
See Day 5 for Recipe

Snack: ¼ cup garlic-roasted almonds or cashew nuts, only if needed

Day 77

Breakfast: Creamy Cream Cheese Flapjacks with Ham and Chives
See Day 8 for Recipe

Lunch: Avocado and Tuna *Ceviche* on *Jicama* Slices
See Day 8 for Recipe

Dinner: Pork Tenderloin Stir-Fry with Cashew Nuts on Zucchini Noodles
See Day 8 for Recipe

Snack: ½ cup fresh berries of choice, only if needed

Day 78

Breakfast: Blueberry and Cashew Milkshake
See Day 2 for Recipe

Lunch: Quick-Pickled Mackerel on Open Faced Cucumber Sandwich
See Day 2 for Recipe

Dinner: Sardine Stuffed Spicy Avocadoes
See Day 2 for Recipe

Snack: ¼ cup shelled pistachio nuts, lightly seasoned, only if needed

Day 79

Breakfast: Almond - Strawberry Milkshake
See Day 4 for recipe

Lunch: Cucumber and Tuna Salad
See Day 4 for recipe

Dinner: Minced Beef Stew on Zucchini Noodles
See Day 1 for recipe

Snack: Hard Boiled Egg, large, lightly seasoned, only if needed

Day 80

Breakfast: Coconut Mushroom Hash
See Day 3 for Recipes

Lunch: Stir-Fried Brussels Sprouts with Bacon on Mung Bean Sprout "Noodles"
See Day 3 for Recipes

Dinner: Minute Pork Chops with Buttered Shiitake Mushrooms
See Day 3 for Recipes

Snack: ¼ cup fried green peas, lightly salted, only if needed

Day 81

Breakfast: Creamy Blueberries in Cream Cheese Flapjacks with Bacon
See Day 5 for Recipe

Lunch: Spicy Sausage Salad with Asparagus
See Day 5 for Recipe

Dinner: Beefy and Spicy Chili
See Day 5 for Recipe

Snack: ¼ cup garlic-roasted almonds or cashew nuts, only if needed

Day 82

Breakfast: Coconut Mushroom Hash
See Day 3 for Recipes

Lunch: Stir-Fried Brussels Sprouts with Bacon on Mung Bean Sprout "Noodles"
See Day 3 for Recipes

Dinner: Minute Pork Chops with Buttered Shiitake Mushrooms
See Day 3 for Recipes

Snack: ¼ cup fried green peas, lightly salted, only if needed

Day 83

Breakfast: Coconut - Mango Milkshake
See Day 1 for recipe

Lunch: Anchovy on Avocado Salad
See Day 1 for recipe

Dinner: Minced Beef Stew on Zucchini Noodles
See Day 1 for recipe

Snack: Hard Boiled Egg, large, lightly seasoned, only if needed

Day 84

Breakfast: Creamy Blueberries in Cream Cheese Flapjacks with Bacon
See Day 5 for Recipe

Lunch: Spicy Sausage Salad with Asparagus
See Day 5 for Recipe

Dinner: Beefy and Spicy Chili
See Day 5 for Recipe

Snack: ¼ cup garlic-roasted almonds or cashew nuts, only if needed

Day 85

Breakfast: Creamy Cream Cheese Flapjacks with Ham and Chives
See Day 8 for Recipe

Lunch: Avocado and Tuna *Ceviche* on *Jicama* Slices
See Day 8 for Recipe

Dinner: Pork Tenderloin Stir-Fry with Cashew Nuts on Zucchini Noodles
See Day 8 for Recipe

Snack: ½ cup fresh berries of choice, only if needed

Day 86

Breakfast: Blueberry and Cashew Milkshake
See Day 2 for Recipe

Lunch: Quick-Pickled Mackerel on Open Faced Cucumber Sandwich
See Day 2 for Recipe

Dinner: Sardine Stuffed Spicy Avocadoes
See Day 2 for Recipe

Snack: ¼ cup shelled pistachio nuts, lightly seasoned, only if needed

Day 87

Breakfast: Coconut Mushroom Hash
See Day 3 for Recipes

Lunch: Stir-Fried Brussels Sprouts with Bacon on Mung Bean Sprout "Noodles"
See Day 3 for Recipes

Dinner: Minute Pork Chops with Buttered Shiitake Mushrooms
See Day 3 for Recipes

Snack: ¼ cup fried green peas, lightly salted, only if needed

Day 88

Breakfast: Blueberry and Cashew Milkshake
See Day 2 for Recipe

Lunch: Quick-Pickled Mackerel on Open Faced Cucumber Sandwich
See Day 2 for Recipe

Dinner: Sardine Stuffed Spicy Avocadoes
See Day 2 for Recipe

Snack: ¼ cup shelled pistachio nuts, lightly seasoned, only if needed

Day 89

Breakfast: Creamy Cream Cheese Flapjacks with Ham and Chives
See Day 8 for Recipe

Lunch: Avocado and Tuna *Ceviche* on *Jicama* Slices
See Day 8 for Recipe

Dinner: Pork Tenderloin Stir-Fry with Cashew Nuts on Zucchini Noodles
See Day 8 for Recipe

Snack: ½ cup fresh berries of choice, only if needed

Day 90

Breakfast: Almond - Strawberry Milkshake
See Day 4 for recipe

Lunch: Cucumber and Tuna Salad
See Day 4 for recipe

Dinner: Minced Beef Stew on Zucchini Noodles
See Day 1 for recipe

Snack: Hard Boiled Egg, large, lightly seasoned, only if needed

Appendix: References / For Further Reading

Online PDF

Davis, E. Fight Cancer with a Ketogenic Diet: A New Method for Treating Cancer. www.ketogenic-diet-resource.com/support-files/rkd-glimpse.pdf

Kenny, L., et. al. Ketogenic Diet: How to Make it Work for Life. www.g1dfoundation.org/wp-content/uploads/2012/01/Ketogenic-Diet-How-to-Make-it-Work-for-Life.pdf

Mercola, D., Ketogenic Diet in Combination with Calorie Restriction and Hyperbaric Treatment Offer New Hope in Quest for Non-Toxic Cancer Treatment. www.oxfordhbot.com/library/cancer/213.021.pdf

McDonald, L. The Ketogenic Diet. www.valetudo.ru/redforum/attachments/9700d1317850791

Neal, E., et. al. The Ketogenic Diet – Classical and MCT. www.site.matthewsfriends.org/uploads/pdf/TypesofKetoDiet.pdf

Phinney, S. Nutrition & Metabolism. Ketogenic Diets and Physical Performance. www.kdheks.gov/nws-wic/download/20-KetogenicDiet.pdf

Schmidt, E., et. al. Effects of a Ketogenic Diet on the Quality of Life in 16 Patients with Advanced Cancer: A Pilot Trial. www.biomedcentral.com/content/pdf/1743-7075-8-54.pdf

Turner, Z., et. al. The Ketogenic and Atkins Diets: Recipes for Seizure Control. http://www.medicine.virginia.edu/clinical/departments/medicin

e/divisions/digestive-health/nutrition-support-team/nutrition-articles/TurnerArticle.pdf

---. An Introduction to the Ketogenic Diet – Continuum of Care. www.coc.unm.edu/common/pdf/Ketodiet_eng_10Dec09.pdf

---. Ketogenic Diet Does Not Affect Strength Performance in Elite Artistic Gymnasts. www.jissn.com/content/pdf/1550-2783-9-34.pdf

Websites

1. www.abcnews.go.com/Health/DiabetesOverview/story?id=38
   43451
2. www.articles.mercola.com/sites/articles/archive/2013/06/16
   /ketogenic-diet-benefits.aspx
3. www.authoritynutrition.com/10-benefits-of-low-carb-
   ketogenic-diets
4. www.diabeticcareservices.com/diabetes-
   education/prediabetes-and-insulin-resistance
5. www.diabetes.co.uk/nutrition/simple-carbs-vs-complex-
   carbs.html
6. www.diabetes.org/living-with-
   diabetes/complications/ketoacidosisdka.html
7. www.diabetes.org/living-with-diabetes/treatment-and-
   care/blood-glucos-control/checking-for-ketones.html
8. www.diagnosisdiet.com/ketogenic-diet-safety/
9. www.drstandley.com/food_whitefood.shtml
10. www.eatingwell.com/nutrition_health/weight_loss_diet_pla
    ns/diet_exercise_tips/6_reasons_you_should_be_eating_ca
    rbs
11. www.examples.yourdictionary.com/examples-of-complex-
    carbohydrates.html
12. www.everydayhealth.com/diet-nutrition/101/nutrition-
    basics/good-carbs-bad-carbs.aspx
13. www.globalhealingcenter.com/natural-health/enriched-
    white-flour/
14. www.healthaliciousness.com/articles/high-omega-3-
    foods.php
15. www.healthline.com/health-news/keto-diet-is-gaining-
    popularity-but-is-it-safe-121914
16. www.healthline.com/health/type-2-diabetes/facts-ketones
17. www.healthline.com/health/inflammatory-bowel-disease
18. www.healthyeating.sfgate.com/foods-contain-white-flour-
    refined-sugars-1330.html

19. www.hhodc.ouhsc.edu/uncategorized/ketoacidosis
20. www.ibreatheimhungry.com/2014/01/week-one-ketolow-carb-7-day-meal-plan-progress.html
21. www.joslin.org/info/ketone_testing_what_you_need_to_know.html
22. www.ketodietapp.com/Blog/post/2015/03/08/Ketogenic-Diet-FAQ-All-You-Need-to-Know
23. www.ketogenic-diet-resource.com/ketogenic-diet-plan.html
24. www.livestrong.com/article/27398-list-complex-carbohydrates-foods/
25. www.lowcarbdoctors.blogspot.com
26. www.mayoclinic.org/diseases-conditions/obesity/basics/complications/con-20014834
27. www.muscleandfitness.com/nutrition/meal-plans/diet-911-ketosis-dummies
28. www.mydreamshape.com/ketogenic-diet-food-list/
29. www.myvmc.com/anatomy/urinary-system-renal-system/
30. www.nhs.uk/Conditions/fatty-liver-disease/Pages/Introduction.aspx
31. www.niddk.nih.gov/health-information/health-topics/Anatomy/your-digestive-system/Pages/anatomy.aspx
32. www.niddk.nih.gov/health-information/health-topics/Diabetes/insulin-resistance-prediabetes/Pages/index.aspx#what
33. www.nlm.nih.gov/medlineplus/ency/imagepages/19534.htm
34. www.nutritionmd.org/nutrition_tips/nutrition_tips_understand_foods/carbs_versus.html
35. www.onegreenplanet.org/vegan-food/benefits-of-complex-carbs-and-the-best-ones-to-eat/
36. www.paleoleap.com/paleo-guide-to-ketosis/
37. www.popsugar.com/fitness/What-Complex-Carbs-35686730
38. www.prevention.com/health/diabetes/what-are-ketones
39. www.ruled.me/30-day-ketogenic-diet-plan
40. www.ruled.me/guide-keto-diet
41. www.study.com/academy/lesson/what-are-macronutrients-definition-functions-examples.html

42. www.sugar-and-sweetener-guide.com/all-sweetener-list.html
43. www.theepochtimes.com/n3/234457-10-foods-that-are-surprisingly-bad-for-you/
44. www.webmd.com/epilepsy/ketogenic-diet-for-epilepsy
45. www.webmd.com/ibd-crohns-disease/crohns-disease/inflammatory-bowel-syndrome

Citations

Adams, M., 2004. Refined Carbohydrates Are to Blame for Skyrocketing Chronic Diseases, Not Just Obesity. Natural News

Bender, D.A., Introduction to Nutrition and Metabolism. 3rd ed. New York, NY: Taylor & Francis, 2002.

Bistrian B.R., et. al. Nitrogen Metabolism and Insulin Requirements in Obese Diabetic Adults on a Protein-Sparing Modified Fast. Diabetes 1976;25:494–504.

Ezrin, C., et. al. The Type II Diabetes Diet Book. Los Angeles, CA: Lowell House, 1995.

Johnston C.S., et.al. Ketogenic Low-Carbohydrate Diets Have No Metabolic Advantage Over Non Ketogenic Low-Carbohydrate Diets. Am J Clin Nutr 2006;83:1055–61.

Levy, R.G., et. al. 2012. Ketogenic Diet and Other Dietary Treatment for Epilepsy. Cochrane Database of Systematic Reviews 3.

Mandel, A., et. al. Medical Costs are Reduced When Children with Intractable Epilepsy are Successfully Treated with the Ketogenic Diet. J Am Diet Assoc 2002;102:396–8.

Neal, E.G., et. al. 2008. The Ketogenic Diet for the Treatment of Childhood Epilepsy: A Randomized Controlled Trial. Lancelot Neurology, 7 (796): 500 – 506.

Wadden, T.A., et.al. <u>Less Food, Less Hunger: Reports of Appetite and Symptoms in a Controlled Study of Protein-Sparing Modified Fast</u>. Int J Obes 1987;11:239–49.

Conclusion

Trying out any new diet can be a challenge as it is, but following a restrictive one poses its own set of problems. This book aims to enlighten you on the basic principle regarding the Ketogenic diet, and how this works as a weight loss option.

This eating regimen is more than just increasing your fat/oil intake. This is a rigorous diet that entails careful planning, careful daily monitoring of your ketone body level, and a solid knowledge on what food/drinks work well for this diet (and which ones you should avoid in the meantime.)

Hopefully, this book will encourage you to follow through with this diet until you achieve ketosis, and ultimately: gradual but safe weight loss.

The next step is to utilize the recipes in this book. If you are confident enough, you can create your own recipes, and adjust the meal plan to suit your personal tastes and lifestyle choices.

Finally, if you find this book informative, can you please give it a 5-star rating?

Thanks again for downloading this book. Good luck on your weight loss endeavor!

Crossfit Diet

The complete guide to getting started with the Crossfit diet

Introduction

I want to thank you and congratulate you for downloading the book, *"Crossfit Diet: The complete guide to getting started with the crossfit diet"*.

This book contains proven steps and strategies on how to get started with the crossfit diet that can effectively provide your body with the right sustenance it needs while you do the workouts. Crossfit training can help you lose weight, enhance your strength and stamina, provides balance, and make you feel good about yourself.

The crossfit workouts are more rigid than your usual exercises, and you will see positive results if you do it on regular basis. To effectively pull it off, you need to eat the right diet that will be able to support your body while training. This book can help you decide for the right foods to eat and succeed in your endeavor.

You also need to have patience, discipline, diligence, and will power to help yourself see the results that you want to see.

Thanks again for downloading this book, I hope you enjoy it!

Chapter 1: Crossfit Diet 101: Understanding What Crossfit is and the Diet that Works

Crossfit is a complete fitness program. Its creator Greg Glassman, a former gymnast, involved a combination of several workouts to come up with the most effective set of exercises for an athlete. The exercises include cardiovascular workouts, functional strength training, and intense athletic movements. The crossfitter needs to give his body the right sustenance it needs to cope up with the rigid exercises that the program requires to give the maximum benefit.

Among the available diet programs around, the Paleo diet works well (and it is the most suitable diet) with the set of exercises that the crossfit program requires. The Paleo diet follows a dietary guideline based on the presumed early diet of the Paleolithic men. This diet requires nuts, vegetables, fruit, fish, and meat (pork, chicken, or beef). It is taboo to include dairy, legumes, grain, and processed food in a Paleo diet – to sum it up, do not eat any kind of food that did not exist during the Paleolithic age.

Every type of food in a Paleo diet is exactly the kind of food that a crossfitter needs to consume. It will give him the right sustenance that can help him with his crossfit training. The Paleo diet can provide the right amount of protein, fiber, and other necessary nutrients that he will need as he trains. But still, you need to modify the Paleo diet in order to fit into your crossfitter life.

Your deeper understanding regarding the foods that you are allowed and not allowed to eat in a Paleo diet can help you plan your meal – something that you and your whole family could share. Your family will surely love the succulent dishes that they won't mind eating the dishes that you prepared while following the protocols in the Paleo diet program. You will learn more about Paleo Diet in Chapter 2, and some of the succulent dishes in Chapter 4.

Advantages of Crossfit Diet Over the other Diet Programs

The required crossfit diet of the crosfitter is the same as the Paleo diet. There should be a lot of protein and other important nutrients. You also need to consume lots of water to replenish the lost liquid during the training or workout.

The Paleo diet is the most ideal diet program to follow when doing crossfit training. You don't need to closely monitor the calories of each food you take, as long as you have the right proportion of food on your plate. You also need to keep in mind the kinds of food that the early men usually eat during the Paleolithic period.

You won't be deprived of flavors when you switch to Paleo diet. There are a lot of recipes that offer succulent dishes that are tailored for Paleo diet. You can serve the same dish to your entire family and get them fit in no time.

There are guilt-free desserts that you can try. Paleo diet uses natural sweeteners to whip up a tasty dessert. You are not permitted to use processed sugar granules, aside from the fact that sugar can bring more harm to your body than good. Some uses Stevia, honey, or molasses when creating their own dessert recipe. Never use artificial sweeteners because they are packed with preservatives that can only harm your body.

When you switch to Paleo diet, you won't feel like you are following a diet program. You can cook anything within the specified list of food that you can eat, and you practically don't need to measure each portion to take. It is easy and simple to follow, and you won't starve.

If you do crossfit training, you need a well fed body to avoid breaking down. The other diet programs tend to make you hungry because you need to burn more calories if you do crossfit workout. If you limit your caloric intake, then there's a huge possibility that your body won't be able to cope. The ideal crossfit diet, the Paleo diet, won't make your body starve and you can work out for long hours. You might need to slightly modify the Paleo diet to fit into your training.

The Crossfit Nutrition

Crossfit has its own dietary guidelines that the crossfitter needs to follow together with the exercises in the crossfit training.

The official CrossFit website says that the needed nutrients should follow this proportion: 40% carbohydrates, 30 % protein, and 30% fat. A crossfitter can get the needed amount of nutrients by eating only vegetables, nuts, lean meats, and seeds. The CrossFit website further states that the diets that are high in carbohydrates have the power to raise a person's insulin levels. An increased insulin level can lead to obesity and occurrence of chronic disease. You can find the complete list of good sources of carbohydrates, protein, and fat on Chapter 2.

The CrossFit organization also believes that a reduced calorie has the ability to promote longevity. It also decreases the risks of having heart disease and/or cancer.

You need to learn to eat only quality foods that your body needs. For most people, this is something hard to do. Those who are used to having bread, grains, and other processed carbohydrates are likely to give up if they can't part with the said foods. But, if you are someone who is determined to succeed in your endeavor, then you need to learn how to control yourself from consuming the taboo foods that the crossfit diet strictly prohibits. You need to shop for lean meats, fruits and vegetables, nuts, and seeds. It is not recommended to switch abruptly to crossfit diet, you can try small changes in your diet each day until you get used to it. Small, regular, and sustained changes are the things that you need to keep in mind when switching to the crossfit diet.

You are Already Eating Quality Foods

If you are accustomed to eating quality foods, the next thing you need to learn is how to get the right proportions of your quality foods that will give you the amount of fuel that you need for your workout. Supplying your body with the right quantity of fuel will prevent breakdown.

It is recommended that you consume the suggested proportions in "The Crossfit Nutrition" section of this book. It is also recommended that you take regular small meals throughout the day.

What about my Family?

To be blunt, you will never hear any complaints from your family about the meal if you can give them something succulent yet won't defy your diet program. Preparing two sets of meal (one for you, and one for the entire family) can invite an argument. Your family might feel alienated when you do that, and they might feel like you are separating yourself from them. It might even create barriers, which you don't want to happen.

If you can suggest recipes that you all can agree on (of course they are Paleo friendly recipes), then the problem will be solved in a matter of time. You need to include your family with certain decisions before you proceed with your plan. There are great recipes in this book that you will all surely agree on.

The earlier you start your kids with Paleo diet, the better. You can be certain that they will grow up healthy and fit, and they will carry that to their adult years. You don't need to worry too much about their health even if they have to part from you and leave home.

When Eating Out

Eating out with family and friends is something inevitable. You don't need to worry about sacrificing your diet or having fun – you can have fun while eating the required proportion in your crossfit diet. You can estimate the quality portion of your protein by using the palm of your hand – your meat should be about that big. You can choose your carbs from the list of fruits and vegetables found on Chapter 2. If you have a palm-sized steak, then you can have broccoli along with your steak.

Drinking Alcohol

Drinking alcohol is not prohibited, and a crosfitter is allowed to drink occasionally. Anything taken excessively, not just alcohol, is bad. There are crossfit athletes who consume alcohol once in a while and there are those who completely abstain from drinking alcohol. Most crossfit atheletes who gain success in their endeavor do not drink alcohol at all. To be frank, if you want to succeed, then it is best to stay away from alcohol.

Aside from the right diet and workout, you need to make sure that your body gets proper rest and you must sleep when it is time to sleep.

Chapter 2: Getting Started with the Crossfit Diet

Earlier, you learned that Paleo is the most ideal diet to follow if you are a crossfitter. This book assumes that you follow a regular regimen for your workout, and you need a suitable diet to meet your goal.

Paleo diet is the closest diet program that can sustain you body with all the needed nutrients and sustenance that it needs to satisfy the demands of the crossfit training. This book can help you modify your Paleo diet to perfectly fit into your crossfitter life. You need to gain a clear understanding regarding the foods that you can eat and not to eat on the Paleo diet. It can help a lot when you plan for your meal. Keep in mind that simplicity is beauty, and it only means that simpler meals are always better than complicated ones.

Your Food Guide

To make Paleo works for you it is important to think like a predator and don't act like a prey. What does that mean? Paleolithic men were meat eaters. You need to effectively mimic that time period, but we will modify it a bit. You are expected to eat organic meats as your protein source, good amount of fats, and some fruits and vegetables for your carbohydrates.

It is advisable to find grass-fed meat in the market if you can. Red meats like venison, bison (the meat source that closely resembles the one in the Paleolithic Age), goat, elk, and beef are the best choices. You can be certain that a grass-fed meat doesn't contain chemicals as compared to meats that were fed with feeds that contain different chemicals. Pork and chicken must be consumed in moderation, the excessive omega-6 they contain make them far less healthy.

It would be easier for you to plan your meal if you have a list of quality sources for your carbohydrates, fats, and protein.

Your Quality Carbohydrates

When you talk about quality carbohydrates you need to think about antioxidants. High quality carbs should be able to provide antioxidants and keeps the insulin and blood sugar levels as steady as possible.

The good sources of quality carbs are as follows:

Class	Food Items
Excellent Source of Carbohydrates	Vegetables:
	Cauliflower
	Broccoli
	Kale
	Romaine lettuce
	Spinach
	Fruits:
	Blackberries
	Blueberries
	Strawberries
Very Good Source of Carbohydrates	Vegetables:
	Cabbage
	Brussels sprouts
	Eggplant
	Onion
	Red pepper
	String beans
	Fruits:
	Kiwi

	Pink Grapefruit
	Plum
	Tomato
Good Source of Carbohydrates	Vegetables:
	Celery
	Cucumber
	Yellow squash
	Fruits:
	Green grapes
	Orange
	Pear
	Red grapes

Your Quality Protein

When you define the quality of a protein of a certain food source, you need to think about its fat content. Understand that all protein food sources, including tofu, have fat.

The good sources of quality protein are as follows:

Class	Food Items
Excellent Source of Protein	Cod
	Haddock
	Lobster
	Mackerel
	Salmon
	Sea bass
	Snapper
	Soybean hamburger crumbles

	Tuna steak
	Turkey breast
	Turkey breast, deli
Very Good Source of Protein	Chicken breast
	Chicken breast, deli
	Cottage cheese (1%)
	Emu
	Freshwater bass
	Trout
	Tuna, canned in water
	Soy imitation meat products
Good Source of Protein	Beef tenderloin, well-trimmed
	Pork tenderloin, well-trimmed
	Tempeh
	Tofu, extra-firm
	Tofu, firm
	Tofu, soft
Low-Quality Source of Protein	Bacon
	Ground beef (27% fat)
	Sausage

Your Quality Fats

You need quality fat to provide better fuel for your body. The best sources of quality fat are the foods that contain high concentration of monounsaturated fats and low in Omega-6 and saturated fats. The saturated fats can raise your cholesterol levels, which usually give heart disease.

The good sources of quality fats are as follows:

Class	Food Items
Excellent Source of Fats	Olives
	Olive oil
	Macadamia nuts
Very Good Quality Source of Fats	Almond butter
	Almonds
	Avocado
	Canola oil
Good Quality Source of Fats	Cashews
	Peanuts
Poor Quality Source of Fats	Butter
	Lard
	Soybean oil
	Safflower oil

If you can come up with a meal plan that includes the best sources of quality barbs, protein, and fats, then choose to do that. However, there are times when your body craves for the food sources that provide lesser benefits (but still considered an okay source of the needed nutrients); you can include them as well just make sure not to do it regularly. You won't be able to get used to eating quality foods if you always include foods that give lesser benefits. Yes, you should not include the foods that won't give any benefit at all.

Also, you need to completely stay away from junk foods, they bring nothing but trouble. It is recommended not to try them anymore, especially if you are already used to eating the recommended food sources.

Chapter 3: Your Very Own Paleo Staples

Preparing a Paleo meal in a jiffy is not always possible, and having a simple Paleo meal might become boring at one point. You might still crave for a more flavorful or fancier dish once in a while. Unfortunately, to make a flavorful dish you need to follow a recipe that is a bit complicated. The good news is you can still whip up a succulent meal within fifteen minutes if you have your basic and/or pre-cooked ingredients ready beforehand.

You can buy the Paleo staples in groceries or supermarkets, but you can't really be sure if you are buying something that is free from chemical preservatives and other ingredients that are not Paleo friendly. The only way to make sure is if you make the staples yourself.

Bone Broth

You can store this homemade bone broth in the freezer. It is recommended to use silicone muffin mold when freezing your broth. Let the broth cool first after making it. When it has cooled, get your silicon mold and carefully pour the broth in each muffin hole. Put the mold in the freezer and wait for it to turn solid. Remove the frozen broth from the mold and store it in Ziploc. The frozen broth is good within seven days.

You can prepare a quick soup using the frozen broth. You simply pop two or more broth blocks in a casserole, and heat the broth over low fire. Bring it to boil, and add some vegetables and pre-cooked meat to make a delightful quick soup.

Use a 6-quart pressure cooker to cook your broth.

Ingredients:

2 leaks, trimmed and halved
2 carrots, peeled and quartered
2.5 pounds of bones (choice of chicken, pork, or beef)
8 cups water
1 teaspoon apple cider vinegar
2 tablespoons salt

Procedure:

1. Put all the ingredients in the pressure cooker, lock it, and set it to high pressure.

2. Cook your ingredients over high heat.

3. Immediately bring down the cooker's temperature once it reached high pressure. Cook for thirty or more minutes.

4. Turn off the stove, and wait for the pressure inside the cooker to naturally release.

5. Strain the broth, and let it cool for a bit.

You can use a slow cooker if you don't have a pressure cooker, but expect it to take longer to cook.

Paleo Mayonnaise

It is good to use Paleo mayonnaise for dishes in your crossfit diet that need mayo. There is a lot of Paleo mayonnaise in the market, but you wouldn't know if the Paleo mayonnaise that you are buying is the real deal. To be safe, make your own Paleo mayonnaise, it's easy.

Ingredients:

2 yolks of organic eggs
Half teaspoon of salt
A pinch of white pepper
1 tablespoon Dijon mustard
2 tablespoons lemon juice
1½ cups macadamia or avocado oil

Procedure:

Use room temperature ingredients.

1. Combine all the ingredients in a steel or ceramic bowl, except oil.

2.   Beat or whip the ingredients until you get a smooth consistency.

3. Add the oil while whisking, make sure to add in thin stream.

4. If the mixture begins to cling to the sides of the bowl, then you can slowly stir in the remaining oil while you continue whisking.

You can store your fresh mayonnaise in the refrigerator to maximum of three days. You can drizzle some of it on your favorite greens after making it, and enjoy a truly guilt-free salad.

These Paleo staples are great help in preparing your Paleo dishes.

Chapter 4: Some Crossfit Recipes to Try

This chapter is dedicated to some of the ideal recipes you can try to start your crossfit diet. You can create different combinations of the dishes as you make a meal plan. There are different healthy dressings that you can try when you are on the go.

Caesar Dressing ala Paleo

The Caesar dressing is versatile enough to add in any salad, and you can use it as dip. You can add other spices to your liking or use it as it is.

Ingredients:

1 tablespoon lemon juice
2 tablespoons Paleo mayo
Half cup of olive oil, extra-virgin
5 cloves of garlic, minced
1 tablespoon Dijon mustard
Anchovy fillets, minced
Some ground black pepper and sea salt to taste

Procedure:

Use your blender to combine garlic, lemon juice, and mustard. Add the mayonnaise and continue blending. Slowly put in the olive oil while the blender keeps on going. After blending, use your spatula to scrape all the finished dressing in a bowl. Season it with salt and pepper; add a bit more of lemon juice together with the anchovy fillet. Taste and adjust.

Vinaigrette: Raspberry-Walnut

This vinaigrette is inspired by lemon vinaigrette. Instead of using lemon juice and olive oil, we will use raspberry vinegar and walnut oil.

Ingredients:

3 tablespoons raspberry vinegar
Half teaspoon of Dijon mustard

3/4 cup walnut oil
Salt and ground black pepper to taste
2 tablespoons walnuts, chopped

Procedure:

Get a bowl and combine all the ingredients, except the chopped walnuts. Adjust the taste before adding the chopped walnuts.

Vinaigrette: Rosemary and Orange

This recipe is also inspired by lemon vinaigrette.

Ingredients:

3 tablespoons fresh lime or lemon juice
Half teaspoon of Dijon mustard
3/4 cup olive oil, extra-virgin
1 orange, get the juice and grate the zest
1 teaspoon rosemary, chopped
Salt and ground black pepper to taste

Procedure:

Get a bowl and mix all the ingredients. Adjust the taste and infuse overnight.

Ginger Vinaigrette Asian Style

This vinaigrette is a good dressing for bitter greens or salads with roasted beets.

Ingredients:

1 large ginger, peeled and grated
3 tablespoons rice vinegar
2/3 cup olive oil, extra-virgin
1 tablespoons sesame oil
Salt and ground black pepper to taste

Procedure:

Squeeze the grated ginger to get 1 tablespoons of juice, discard the ginger after getting the juice. Combine the ginger juice and rice vinegar in a bowl. While whisking the ingredients in the bowl, add olive oil a little at a time. Put in the sesame oil and season to taste.

Classic Pan Seared Steak

It's impossible to go wrong with this pan seared steak. It is easy to prepare, succulent, and guilt-free. This is good for four persons.

Ingredients:

4 grass-fed rib eye steaks, about 10 ounces and 1-inch thick each
dry rub (combine: 2 teaspoons salt, 1 finely chopped onion, 2 teaspoons black pepper, 2 cloves minced garlic, 1 teaspoon paprika)
4 sprigs of rosemary
4 tablespoons clarified butter
1 whole garlic, peeled and minced
Coconut oil

Procedure:

1. Brush your room temperature steaks with some coconut oil to prevent the dry rub from escaping.

2. Coat each steak with the dry rub.

3. Set aside. Allow the meat to absorb the flavors of the dry rub.

4. Ready your cast iron pan and put it over high heat. When you see smoke, your pan is ready.

5. Put your steaks in the pan, and cook each side for 3 minutes for medium rare. You need to cook longer if you want it well done.

6. Set the cooked steaks aside, keep them warm by covering them with foil.

7. Put a pan over medium low heat, and add the steak drippings, butter, garlic cloves, and rosemary. Slightly brown the garlic, and

when the fragrance of rosemary fills the air you can turn off the heat and pour it over your steaks.

Serve your dish and enjoy.

Stir Fried Ground Beef with Cabbage

This recipe serves two to three people.

Ingredients:

2 pounds ground beef (preferably grass-fed)
1 cup water chestnuts, sliced
1 head Napa cabbage, julienned
3 cloves garlic, minced
1 clove garlic, minced
1/2 cup bamboo shoots, julienned
1 tablespoon fresh ginger root, julienne cut
3/4 cup coconut aminos
1/2 cup scallions thinly cut
2 tablespoons sesame seeds
Pinch of black pepper
2-3 tablespoons coconut oil

Procedure:

1. Get two pans – for the ground beef and the cabbage.

2. Put each pan on separate burners over medium heat.

3. Put 2 tablespoons oil in the ground beef pan and 1 tablespoon oil in the other pan.

4. You can now add the beef in the ground beef pan, and turn the beef occasionally as it cooks.

5. You can also add the cabbage in the other pan. Toss it until the oil covers the cabbage. Let it wilt.

6. Add the ginger over the half done beef, followed by bamboo shoots and water chestnuts.

7. Add 1 clove minced garlic on the other pan when you see that the volume has reduced. Coat the cabbage with garlic by tossing.

8. Add 3 cloves minced garlic in the beef pan. Slightly brown the beef.

9. Add 1/4 cup coconut aminos on the cabbage and reduce it a bit before serving.

10. In the ground beef pan, add in 1/2 cup coconut aminos, black pepper, and sesame seeds. Let the aminos reduce a bit.

11. You can remove either pan (or both pans) from heat after reducing the coconut aminos.

All-Time Favorite Meatballs

This recipe will yield around 18 meatballs.

Ingredients:

1 pound ground beef
4 pieces shiitake mushrooms, finely chopped
1/3 cup boiled sweet potatoes, mashed
1 tablespoon cilantro, finely chopped
1 small shallot, finely chopped
1 tablespoon tomato paste
Salt and pepper to taste
1 tablespoon coconut oil

Procedure:

1. Preheat the oven to 375°F.

2. Line your baking sheet with aluminum foil, and brush it with coconut oil.

3. Get a large bowl and toss the mushrooms, shallot, sweet potato, and cilantro in there.

4. You then add the ground beef, salt, pepper, and tomato paste.

5. Mix everything in the bowl well.

6. Form balls that measure 1 to 1 ½ inch in diameter.

7. Neatly arrange the finished meatballs on the baking sheet. Bake the meatballs for 10 to 15 minutes. You need to rotate the tray once in a while to ensure even cooking.

After baking, you can serve the meatballs or store them in your refrigerator after they have cooled.

Quick Pan Roasted Chicken

This recipe is quick and easy to prepare, and it is good for two people.

Ingredients:

3 large chicken thighs, halved
3 sprigs of thyme
A pinch of black pepper
1/2 teaspoon sea salt, finely ground
1/2 cup bone broth (whatever you have) with a splash of balsamic vinegar

Procedure:

1. Preheat the oven to 450°F.

2. Combine the sea salt and pepper – this will serve as your rub for your chicken thighs.

3. Get your oven-safe skillet, and put it over medium heat.

4. Sear the chicken pieces, skin touching the skillet, for three to five minutes.

5. When the chicken skin turned brown (not burnt), reverse the pieces and cook the other side for two minutes.

6. Add the broth and sprigs of thyme, and then put the skillet in the oven. Let the chicken roast for ten minutes or until tender.

Serve your dish and enjoy your meal.

Classic Chicken Liver Pâté

This recipe is easy to do, and you would want to savor it time and again.

Ingredients:

Half pound chicken livers
1 clove garlic, minced
3 slices of bacon, cubed
3 tablespoons sherry or vinegar
1 onion, diced
3/4 cup clarified butter
4 tablespoons parsley, chopped
Salt and pepper to season
Fresh nutmeg (optional)

Procedure:

1. Put the bacon on a large pan and cook over medium heat for three minutes.

2. Add in the garlic, onion, and 1/4 cup butter. Cook for another three to four minutes.

3. Prepare the chicken livers, remove the stringy part.

4. Put the livers to the pan and cook for 7 to 10 minutes. Add some more butter.

5. Add sherry, fresh nutmeg, parsley, salt, and pepper. Taste and adjust if needed.

6. Remove from heat and pour in a blender and blend until it reached a smooth consistency.

7. Pour the mixture in a dish.

8. Melt the remaining butter and evenly spread on the pâté.

9. Cover and keep in the refrigerator to cool, and to harden the fat.

You can also enjoy this pâté as a snack.

Paleo Coco-Vanilla Ice Cream

Yes, you can make a guilt-free ice cream to enjoy.

Ingredients:

1 can coconut milk, full-fat
4 egg yolks
4 tablespoons vanilla extract

Flavoring options:

your choice of berries, chopped or pureed
coconut flakes
chopped mint
chopped nuts
lemon, orange, or lime zest
raw honey
dark chocolate chips or flakes

Procedure:

1. Get a pot and boil some water, and then reduce the heat to simmer.

2. Create a double boiler by putting a heat proof bowl over it. Pour the coconut milk in the heat proof bowl. Add the vanilla extract, and heat it, but don't make it boil. If you choose to add mint or dark chocolate, it is the right time to add them now.

3. Get a separate bowl to whisk the egg yolks. Continue whisking the egg as you add the hot coconut milk by ladleful while keeping the eggs from being cooked in the hot coconut milk.

4. Pour the egg mixture into the double boiler, continue whisking.

5. Keep on whisking non-stop until you see a thick custard begins to form. Don't let it get too hot, and the simmering water must not touch the mixture.

6. When the custard is ready, you can now remove it from heat and let it cool on the table before you put it in the refrigerator.

7. You can add more flavoring later when the custard becomes cold enough to stick your finger in it.

8. Cool it more in the refrigerator, then put in the freezer.

9. Get your ice cream maker, follow its instructions, let your ice cream set. You can also try to put it in a baking dish, and take it out from the freezer to stir vigorously every 30 minutes. Do it for about 2 to 3 hours.

Enjoy your homemade guilt-free ice cream.

Quick Blueberry Dump Cake

This recipe is a must-try.

Ingredients:

1 pack Paleo-friendly yellow cake mix
1 teaspoon cinnamon, ground
1 cup coconut milk
Half cup ghee, melted
4 cups blueberries
Half cup coconut sugar

Procedure:

1. Preheat the oven to 350°F.

2. Get a baking dish and mix cinnamon, berries, and coconut sugar.

3. Get a bowl and put in the yellow cake mix and add coconut milk, mix them well.

4. Pour the yellow cake mixture over the berries, and pour ghee over the yellow cake mix without mixing.

6. Bake for 30 minutes or until slightly brown.

Let it cool before serving.

Fried Fish Curry

Ingredients:

2 pounds fillet of white fish
2 teaspoons curry powder
4 organic egg yolks
1/4 teaspoon pepper
1 teaspoon cumin
1 cup coconut, shredded
1 teaspoon salt
Lemon zest
Coconut oil

Procedure:

1. Make sure that your fish fillet is dry. Use a towel if you need to dry it.

2. Get a pan and put it over medium heat.

3. Add the coconut oil when the pan is hot enough, and make sure to cover the entire fish fillet.

4. As you wait for the cooking oil to get hot, get a bowl and whip the egg yolks.

5. Get a separate bowl, and add in the spices and coconut. Mix everything well.

6. Cover each fish fillet with egg, and then coat it with the coconut mixture.

7. Test if the oil is hot before deep frying the fish. Cook the fish until it turns golden brown.

Bacon, Mush, and Spinach

This dish is amazingly delicious that you might find it hard to believe that it's so simple to prepare.

Ingredients:

1 pound smoked bacon, cut into bite size strips
Half pound of button mushrooms, cut into four
2 cloves garlic, minced
2 handfuls of spinach, cut off the stems
1 onion, coarsely chopped
1 tablespoon lard
Dash of salt and pepper to taste

Procedure:

1. Get a casserole and put it over medium heat.

2. Add in the bacon, and let it release its natural fat. It is important not to make the bacon crispy.

3. Add the garlic, onion, and mushroom. Cook until the mushroom becomes tender.

4. Add spinach and lard.

7. Cover your casserole. Stir it occasionally, and cook until the spinach becomes tender.

8. Season it with salt and pepper. Serve.

Sweet Potato Fries Recipe

Ingredients:

2 pounds sweet potatoes, cut in wedges
1/4 cup coconut oil
2 to 3 teaspoons fresh or dried herb of your choice
Salt and pepper to season

Procedure:

1. Preheat the oven to 425°F.

2. Get a bowl and add in the oil and herbs. Add in the potato wedges and coat each piece with oil and herb mixture.

3. Add salt and pepper to season.

4. Align the wedges on a baking tray to cook evenly.

5. Cook the potato wedges for about 20 minutes.

6. Prick the wedges with the tip of your knife and see if they are tender enough to eat. If not, you need to cook them in the oven for another 5 minutes, and then test again.

Serve your sweet potato wedges and enjoy.

You can create simple soups with your frozen broth by adding your choice of vegetables and pre-cooked meat. You can also use the frozen broth for a tastier dish. You can mix and match the dishes in this chapter in planning your meal. You and your family will get to enjoy a healthy and great tasting meal all the time.

Chapter 5: Common Mistakes in Meal Planning for Crossfit Diet

Although Paleo diet is the most ideal diet program for a crossfitter to follow, you still need to modify it to meet the nutritional requirements of your body. Paleo could teach you how to eat clean and quality foods all the time. You can turn it into a habit in the long run.

Strictly Follows a Paleo Diet

If you are a crossfitter that does it for recreational purposes, then following a Paleo diet can give you a healthy and fit body without trouble. However, it is different if you are an athlete who intends to compete. If you are training rigidly for more than two hours a day, then your main source of energy is quality carbohydrates. The usual Paleo Diet does not provide enough carbohydrates to properly support your training. Even so, it does not mean you have to stuff your tummy with bread, sugar, and pasta just to get the carbohydrates that your body needs. Don't forget that you must consume quality carbohydrates (refer to the food guide list) as much as possible.

You can add "other" carbohydrates once in a while, but make sure that you have enough will power to stop yourself from craving too much bad carbohydrates. Sugar is definitely an enemy that you need to stay away from.

Finds it Hard to Believe that Diet Alone won't Do

Your diet plays a crucial role in providing your body with the right amount of nutrients it needs to support you during intense workouts. But, diet is not the only thing responsible for attaining success in your endeavor. Everything must be balanced. You need to have the right amount of exercise, the right foods, proper rest, healthy recreational activities, and other factors. You should not rely on your diet alone to give you the results that you want to see.

A Well Planned Diet Gives Faster Results

There are some people who spend so much time planning for the most ideal diet that could give them the results they want to see in just a few weeks. However, when they failed to see it most of them get frustrated and eventually stop doing the training and diet program all together.

Know that even if you have a well planned diet, you will not see a large impact within a few weeks. Your body is slowly changing from deep within, and you will not see it until after some months.

Create a well planned diet if you want, but don't expect to see immediate results. Don't stop doing what you have started just because you failed to see the expected results that you want to see within the time frame that you set. The moment you stop doing it, your body will only go back to the way it was before, and any initial improvement that already happened deep within will no longer manifest on the surface.

Plan a Meal that's Right for the Needs of your Body

When you plan your meal, make sure that you have enough of everything to give your body the nutrients it needs during the training. Don't create too much body fuel that you won't be able to burn, and don't deprive your body of the needed fuel when you have rigid workout. Eat the right amount of food with right proportion depending on the kind of training that you intend to do.

It might be a bit tricky to create the correct diet meal plan at first, but soon you will be able to discover the most efficient way of doing it. Also, don't forget to drink plenty of water to keep you hydrated.

Chapter 6: Sample Meal Plan

Below is a sample meal plan that you can try to get you started with your crossfit diet, you can modify it and add more carbohydrates if you train everyday for more than an hour:

	Breakfast	Lunch	Dinner	Snack
Mon	Berries and mixed nuts with coconut milk	Egg salad filled lettuce	Bacon, Mush, and Spinach	Macadamia nuts
Tues	Leftover Bacon, Mush, and Spinach	Chicken broth with veggies and liver pâté	Pan Seared Steak with roasted veggies	Beef jerky
Wed	Spinach omelet and onion with leftover liver pâté	Tuna salad in lettuce with almonds	Beef recipe with Coconut ice cream for dessert	Eggs (Hard boiled)
Thurs	Bacon and eggs with any kind of fruit	Beef recipe and Sweet Potato Wedges	Grilled trout and Paleo broth with some veggies	Smoked salmon
Fri	Smoothie (Coconut milk)	Stir Fried Ground Beef with Cabbage	Roasted chicken with fries (sweet potato)	Almonds and berries mix in a bowl
Sat	Roast chicken (Cold Leftover) with Paleo mayo	Meat balls and Coconut ice cream dessert	Fried Fish Curry and Blueberry Dump Cake	Can of salmon with olive oil & lemon juice
Sun	Stir-fry (Tomato and egg)	Fried pork chops with sautéed spinach	Chicken recipe	Olives & sauerkraut

Chapter 7: Hungry for more Information?

Here are some of the sites that can help you plan your meal, and other things that you need to know about crossfit.

For more recipes that you can include in your diet plan you can visit this site:

http://paleoleap.com/

If you want to know more about how to start a crossfit workout or training, then you can visit this site:

http://www.bodybuilding.com/fun/crossfit-q-a-your-guide-to-starting-crossfit.html

For your ingredients, it is best to visit stores that sell organic produce. Stay away from canned goods that contain chemical preservatives as much as possible. If you want to know more meal planning and the shopping list that you need to have, then you can visit this site:

http://crossfitlongbeach.com/meal-plan-shopping-list

You can have further reading if you go to this site:

http://theathleticbuild.com/diet-of-a-crossfit-athlete/

Start your crossfit diet now, and you will be glad that you did.

Conclusion

Thank you again for downloading this book!

I hope this book was able to help you to create the perfect crosfitter diet plan for yourself.

The next step is to continue practicing what you have learned from this book, and hopefully you will be able to influence your peers to do the same.

Finally, if you enjoyed this book, then I'd like to ask you for a favor, would you be kind enough to leave a review for this book on Amazon? It'd be greatly appreciated!

Click here to leave a review for this book on Amazon!

Thank you and good luck!

www.ingramcontent.com/pod-product-compliance
Lightning Source LLC
Chambersburg PA
CBHW072133280526
45788CB00002B/617